Conducting Systematic Reviews in S
and Physical Activity

David Tod

Conducting Systematic Reviews in Sport, Exercise, and Physical Activity

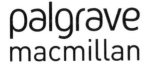

David Tod
School of Sport and Exercise Science
Liverpool John Moores University
Liverpool, UK

ISBN 978-3-030-12262-1   ISBN 978-3-030-12263-8   (eBook)
https://doi.org/10.1007/978-3-030-12263-8

Library of Congress Control Number: 2019932953

This Palgrave Macmillan imprint is published by the registered company Springer Nature
Switzerland AG
The registered company address is: Gewerbestrasse 11, 6330 Cham, Switzerland

Acknowledgements

I would like to thank Grace Jackson, Joanna O'Neill, and Sooryadeepth Jayakrishnan from Palgrave for accepting my idea and their advice. Thanks also to Geoff Bates for his thoughtful comments on earlier drafts of this book. Thank you to Rachel Tod for helping me finish.

Contents

1   Introducing Systematic Reviews 1

2   Planning a Review 17

3   Defining Suitable Review Questions 31

4   Justifying the Review 43

5   Inclusion and Exclusion Criteria 55

6   Undertaking Search Strategies 67

7   Data Extraction 83

8   Critical Appraisal 99

9   Data Analysis and Synthesis 115

10 Assessing the Systematic Review 131

11 Disseminating Results 147

12 Topics Related to Managing a Review 163

13 Top Tips from the Experts 177

    Supplementary Information
    Index 187

List of Figures

Fig. 1.1　Number of SPORTDiscus hits from the search "meta-analysis or systematic review in title". 6

Fig. 2.1　Phases in a systematic review 19

Fig. 2.2　A competency profiling worksheet 26

Fig. 4.1　Creswell's (2014) deficiencies model for an introduction 47

Fig. 6.1　Phases involved in a literature search 69

Fig. 7.1　Example logic model for Langer (2015) 93

Fig. 10.1　Overview of the GRADE procedures 137

Fig. 11.1　The Economic and Social Research Council's steps in developing impact 151

Fig. 12.1　Amount of data at each stage of Tod and Edward's (2015) review 167

List of Tables

Table 1.1   Examples of systematic review types 8
Table 1.2   Examples of review methods suitable for synthesizing
              qualitative evidence 9
Table 2.1   Content of a PRISMA-P protocol (Moher et al., 2015) 23
Table 6.1   Example electronic databases 70
Table 6.2   Items from PRISMA checklist related to search
              documentation 78
Table 7.1   Example items for an extraction form.................... 86
Table 7.2   Example evidence table................................. 92
Table 8.1   Common types of research in sport, exercise,
              and physical activity 104
Table 9.1   Framing a review project............................... 117
Table 9.2   Questions to assist mixed method review design 126
Table 10.1   Topics included in AMSTAR-2 134
Table 10.2   GRADE summary of findings for muscular obsession
              and health behaviours 139
Table 11.1   MOOSE checklist applied to Arcelus et al.'s (2014)
              meta-analysis.. 159
Table 12.1   Stages in a systematic review for which systematic
              review toolbox lists possible information technology
              software... 168
Table 12.2   Garner et al.'s (2016) three step set of questions
              for updating a review 171

Introducing Systematic Reviews

© The Author(s) 2019
D. Tod, *Conducting Systematic Reviews in Sport, Exercise, and Physical Activity*,
https://doi.org/10.1007/978-3-030-12263-8_1

1

Learning Objectives

After reading this chapter, you should be able to:
- Define terms such as systematic review and meta-analysis.
- Describe differences between "black box" and systematic reviews.
- Outline benefits of undertaking systematic reviews.
- Situate systematic reviews within an historical perspective.
- Appreciate the diversity of systematic reviews in sport, exercise, and physical activity.

Introduction

Combine 15 needles in a large concrete mixer along with 50 million straws of hay, and then pile them in a paddock. Now ask friends to find the needles and observe their reactions. The description illustrates the challenges facing people synthesizing research. Estimates indicate more than 50 million scientific publications exist with another 2.5 million being published per year (Ware & Mabe, 2015). Further, 15 studies, on average, are included in a systematic review (Page et al., 2016). Given these figures, the thought experiment above is not farfetched. Fortunately, however, research is not randomly scattered; for example, journals typically focus on specific disciplines which tends to gather together studies of a similar ilk. Nevertheless, given the various ways to disseminate data and the number of studies available, it can be daunting to undertake a systematic review, particularly in the multidisciplinary fields that the sport, exercise, and physical activity umbrellas embrace. To illustrate, I keep a database of research that has measured the drive for muscularity, which first starting appearing in the year 2000 (Edwards & Launder, 2000; McCreary & Sasse, 2000). The database currently holds 330 empirical studies, averaging 19.4 per year. Indicating the accelerating growth, 50% have been produced since 2014, meaning that currently 43 studies are being published each year. These studies have appeared across 71 journals and 87 postgraduate theses, although 39% are located in just 6 periodicals. It takes me considerable time to stay current, yet drive for muscularity is a niche area. The amount of energy and time needed to stay on top of the larger research areas in our fields requires substantially greater investment. My purpose in this book is to dismantle that challenge into its components so that you can make sense of, appreciate, and conduct a systematic review. In this chapter, I set the scene by describing what systematic reviews are and the contributions they make to our fields.

Defining Systematic Reviews

A systematic review:

» Attempts to collate all empirical evidence that fits pre-specified eligibility criteria in order to answer a specific research question. It uses explicit, systematic methods that are selected with a view to minimizing bias, thus providing more reliable findings from which conclusions can be drawn and decisions made. (Chandler, Higgins, Deeks, Davenport, & Clarke, 2017, p. 5)

Key features include (Chandler et al.): (a) clearly stated objectives; (b) pre-defined eligibility criteria; (c) explicit and reproducible methodology; (d) systematic searches to identify all studies meeting the eligibility criteria; (e) assessment of included studies' design quality; (f) evaluation of the validity of the included studies' findings; and (g) systematic presentation and synthesis of the included studies.

Sometimes people confuse systematic reviews with meta-analyses, but they are different beasts (Tod & Eubank, 2017). Meta-analysis involves the use of statistical procedures to synthesize the results from a set of studies. Meta-analytic techniques can be applied to any set of investigations, including those collected unsystematically, in which case the results will be biased. Systematic reviews need not use statistical procedures to integrate findings. The absence (or presence) of meta-analyses does not indicate the quality or usefulness of a systematic review. Both qualitative and quantitative investigations may be included in a research synthesis. Furthermore, high quality meta-analyses will be conducted on studies located via methodical rigorous means.

To help advertise the strengths of systematic reviews, authors pit them against narrative reviews, which they paint as the poor cousins in the synthesis family. The implication is that narrative reviews are unsystematic and of less value than those that synthesize research numerically. Such binary descriptions are misleading, because narrative reviews (where research is synthesized qualitatively) can adhere to Chandler et al.'s (2017) key features. All literature reviews should be underpinned by a systematic approach; otherwise they risk being unduly biased or even little more than opinion pieces (Booth, Sutton, & Papaioannou, 2016). The evaluation of whether a document can, or cannot, be labelled a systematic review does not depend on either the type of evidence included or the use of quantitative over qualitative analysis. Instead, literature reviews can be placed along a continuum from those where authors have adhered to the above features to those where reviewers have stuck loosely, if at all, to them (and have produced "black box" reviews).

Black Box to Systematic Review Continuum

To understand differences between the two review types, I find it helpful to consider systematic reviews as being somewhat similar to primary research (Gough, Oliver, & Thomas, 2017), where the sample consists of research reports instead of people. Some characteristics of good primary research include (a) identifying a relevant, justifiable, and answerable question; (b) employing a reproducible method; (c) being transparent, to allow an external evaluation of the work; and (d) adherence to ethical standards. These characteristics echo those by which Chandler et al. (2017) described systematic reviews. Primary research varies in the degree to which it satisfies these characteristics. For example, it is difficult sometimes to achieve transparency, given journal space limitations, variation in audience understanding, and the difficulty in reducing some procedures to a list of technical steps (Hammersley, 2006). Informed readers realize that all studies have limitations and weigh these against the findings to decide on the investigations' knowledge contributions. Similarly, systematic reviews vary in their adherence to the above characteristics, but that does not make them unsystematic or invalidates their contribution. Again, readers need to evaluate the document in question and decide on the review's usefulness for their needs.

Systematic Review Benefits

Systematic reviews in sport, exercise, and physical activity are similar to other scientific publications in the field: they are written for an audience, including fellow academics, practitioners, and policymakers. Considering the targeted audiences' needs and preferences will help researchers pinpoint their reviews' purposes and justifications. The benefits of undertaking systematic reviews can be classed as knowledge or decision-making support (Pope, Mays, & Popay, 2007).

Knowledge support   A valuable feature of reviews is the synthesis of primary documents. The Cambridge dictionary defines synthesis as "*the mixing of things to make a whole that is different or new*," and this description signals what systematic reviews can achieve. A meta-analysis, for example, "mixes" or combines individual effect sizes to produce a new estimate, along with confidence intervals indicating the range of plausible alternatives to help evaluate the new result. Systematic reviews advance knowledge by informing us about what we know, what we do not know, what we need to know, and why we need to know it. Also, these projects describe the quality of the evidence, allowing us to assess how much confidence we have in what we think we know. More specifically, they allow us to critique evidence and question primary research findings.

Decision-making support   Systematic syntheses can inform audiences about a topic area so they can make evidence-based decisions and policies. When contemplating how to intervene in people's lives, such as implementing exercise adoption programmes, systematic reviews can outline what actions are possible, what actions are not possible, the associated costs and risks, and the potential benefits. By providing support for decision-making processes, systematic reviews may have a real-world impact. For example, systematic reviews often influence the development of public health policy and health-related recommendations proposed by the United Kingdom's National Institute of Clinical Excellence (NICE), as illustrated in their recent evaluation of exercise referral schemes (NICE, 2014).

Typically, primary research is unable to deliver on the above benefits as well as systematic reviews. Individual studies are often localized in their scope and context (Gough et al., 2017). Also, their results may arise through chance or be invalid due to methodological errors, two aspects research syntheses help overcome. In light of these benefits, it is unsurprising that systematic reviews of experimental research sit at the apex of the positivistic hierarchy of evidence that dominates research in many sport, exercise, and physical activity sub-disciplines.

An Historical Narrative

Systematic approaches to reviewing literature are not recent inventions, with some authors identifying landmark examples from the 1700s (Chalmers, Hedges, & Cooper, 2002). Pope et al.'s (2007) description of first and second generation literature reviews reflects one common perspective on the emergence of the modern systematic review.

First generation reviews Literature reviews are an established part of the research industry traceable back to the eighteenth century, although humans have attempted to document and synthesize knowledge for thousands of years (Booth et al., 2016). Booth et al.'s (p. 19) recipe for the traditional literature review illustrates a common way first generation reviews are portrayed: *"take a simmering topic, extract the juice of an argument, add the essence of one filing cabinet, sprinkle liberally with your own publications and shift out the work of noted detractors or adversaries."* The narrative in these portrayals is that first generation reviewers did not focus on addressing answerable questions, provided inadequate explanation of how they undertook their reviews, gave insufficient attention to evaluating the quality of the work they were examining, and (sometimes deliberately) painted biased maps of the landscapes they were surveying. In some cases these criticisms are accurate and authors have produced reviews that would be judged as poor against Chandler et al.'s key features above (Mulrow, 1987; Oxman & Guyatt, 1993; Sacks, Berrier, Reitman, Ancona-Berk, & Chalmers, 1987). It is misleading, however, to lump all traditional reviews in the same basket. There have been first generation or black box review authors who have adopted systematic approaches to their work, but have not reported those methods. They have produced worthwhile documents that have lived long and fruitful lives (Hammersley, 2006). Also, sometimes authors did not aim to provide a systematic review-type summary of the research and their work has still been influential. Just as it is unsuitable to use quantitative criteria to evaluate qualitative research, it is unfitting to apply systematic review standards to documents authors did not intend to be systematic reviews.

Second generation reviews Pope et al. (2007) wrote that a second generation of literature review has been born in which authors adopt systematic synthesis tenets to varying degrees. These reviews are transparent and explicit in their search, analysis, and synthesis of literature. The authors also evaluate the quality of the evidence they are examining, and they *"move beyond a thin description of the evidence to produce higher order syntheses resulting in the production of new knowledge and/or theory"* (p. 6).

In the medical and health-related sciences, the emergence of second generation or systematic reviews has been associated with the rise of the evidence-based movement (Chalmers et al., 2002; Pope et al., 2007). Archie Cochrane is often cited as influential in the development of evidence-based medicine. Cochrane (1972, 1979) argued that much medical practice was ineffective and even harmful, because it was underpinned by inadequate evidence. In a description foreshadowing modern versions of the hierarchy of evidence, Cochrane distinguished between clinical opinion, observational or descriptive studies, and experiments. He advocated the randomized controlled trial (RCT) as the method of choice in guiding medical practice. He also criticized the medical profession, saying *"it is surely a great criticism of our profession that we have not organised a critical summary by speciality or sub-speciality, up-dated periodically, of all relevant RCTS"* (1979, p. 9). Cochrane was the inspiration for the Cochrane Collaboration (Chandler et al., 2017), a non-profit organization focused on organizing medical research findings to support evidence-based healthcare. Its primary function is the preparation and maintenance of systematic reviews.

1

The first and second generation analogy does not reflect a strict chronological timeline. The attempt to adopt systematic approaches to research synthesis has a long history and has not been confined to (or even emerged solely from) the medical and health-related fields (Chalmers et al., 2002). Although earlier attempts to be systematic may look different to those undertaken today, there has been a long line of reviewers who approached research synthesis in methodical and transparent ways. These reviewers have attempted to meet two key challenges: finding ways to increase precision in synthesis and to minimize potential biases in the review process (Chalmers et al.).

A third generation? If the medical and health fields are latecomers to the systematic review nightclub (Chalmers et al., 2002), then many disciplines in the sport, physical activity, and exercise fields are still talking to the bouncers, but there are signs that systematic reviews are becoming more popular in our literature base. ▣ Figure 1.1, for example, presents the results by year of an unsophisticated search of SPORTDiscus using the keywords "systematic review" or "meta-analysis" in the title. The graph reveals that the number of hits returned per year has been increasing rapidly since the early 2000s. The results reflect the suggestion of an accelerating production of systematic reviews.

One reason for the accelerating output is probably the increased numbers of researchers and academics in the field. Sport, exercise, and physical activity-related fields have experienced considerable growth over the last 30–40 years. The sheer weight of numbers, however, is probably not enough to explain the rapid increase. Historically, academics have considered reviewing research as "*second-class scientifically derivative work … characterized as 'parasitic recycling' of the work of those engaged in the real business of science*" (Chalmers et al., 2002, pp. 21–22). Such a perception has changed in recent years. One stimulus for the attitude change may be the influence of funders,

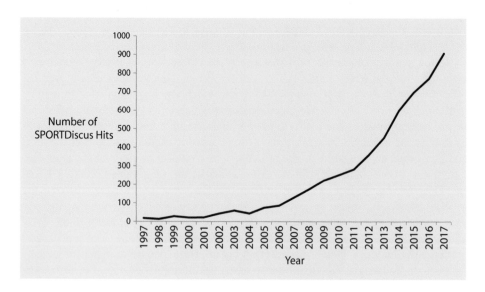

▣ **Fig. 1.1**   Number of SPORTDiscus hits from the search "meta-analysis or systematic review in title"

policymakers, and research consumers. Primary research typically focuses on a narrow question (e.g., how much does physical activity influence obesity levels in children?). Stakeholders want answers to questions not normally suited to individual studies, but involve an accumulation of evidence from multiple projects across several disciplines (e.g., should public money be used to promote physical activity among children?). Stakeholders may find systematic reviews more helpful than primary research. If the people who fund and consume research start asking for reviews, then their perceived value in academia will rise. Along a related line, researchers are increasingly held accountable for their productivity, as shown in the government-led research assessment exercises in countries such as the UK, Australia, and New Zealand. Metrics, such as citation rates, the H-index, and journal impact factors, represent one way to assess productivity. Systematic reviews can often garner higher metrics than primary research.

Another reason for the increase in published research syntheses could be the wide variety of ways reviews may be undertaken. Academics have largely overcome the myth that research synthesis is confined to the aggregation of statistical findings from intervention studies (Petticrew, 2001). Research synthesis reflects a process that can be applied to various evidence types. Further, the process needs to be tailored to suit the purposes and questions under examination: one size does not fit all. Particularly given the acceptance of qualitative research, reviewers have devoted attention to finding ways to synthesize evidence of various types. Reviewers can choose an approach that suits their needs from a range of methods, as illustrated next.

Systematic Review Diversity in Sport, Exercise, and Physical Activity

Creativity is a feature of high quality reviews, such as knowing how to adapt the process to specific questions. Authors' latitude, however, does not mean anarchy rules. There are criteria by which to guide and evaluate systematic reviews, including transparency, precision, and reproducibility. Also, authors do not have to start from ground zero, and there are various types of reviews already well established from which investigators can select a method suited to their purposes. ◼ Tables 1.1 and 1.2 illustrate the variation in reviews. These tables are not exhaustive, but list some popular approaches used in sport, exercise, and physical activity.

◼ Table 1.1 begins with scoping and mapping reviews which may sometimes be quicker to complete and involve less synthesis and critical appraisal sophistication than traditional systematic reviews. Meta-analyses and the Cochrane style review represent gold standard methods. Economic evaluations are a relatively new addition to the genre in sport, exercise, and physical activity, but given that money for public interventions is typically limited, the frequency of these reviews is likely to blossom. As systematic reviews have become recognized as legitimate forms of research (Chalmers et al., 2002), umbrella reviews or overviews, defined as reviews of reviews, have emerged. Ioannidis (2016) estimates that in some topic areas more reviews than primary research are being published annually. Also, frequently the findings of these overlapping reviews conflict with each other. Umbrella reviews help professionals make sense of the information emerging from multiple systematic reviews.

1

□ Table 1.1   Examples of systematic review types

Review type	Definition	Example
Scoping review	Initial estimation of size and scope of evidence, typically designed to help with planning of future reviews or research. Exhaustive searching or critical appraisal often absent	Stork and colleagues' (2017) scoping review of psychological responses to interval exercise
Mapping review	Categorizes existing evidence by design, variables examined, or other attributes relevant to stakeholder needs. Exhaustive search possible, but often no critical appraisal. Typically designed to help with future review planning, but may be publishable itself	Langer' (2015) mapping review on sport-for-development's effectiveness in Africa
Meta-analysis	Uses statistical techniques to gain numerical answers to specific questions. Ideally searches are exhaustive and critical appraisal results are used to further understanding (e.g., sensitivity or moderation analysis)	Macnamara and colleagues' (2016) review of the deliberate practice and sport performance relationship
Cochrane-style review	A review conforming to the Cochrane Collaboration's guidelines. Searches are exhaustive and extensive critical appraisal undertaken. Historically focused on meta-analysis of randomized controlled trials	Martin and colleagues' (2018) review on the effects of physical activity, diet, and other behavioural interventions on cognition and school achievement in overweight or obese children and adolescents
Economic evaluation review	Systematic review of economic evaluations of intervention cost effectiveness, often compared with rival strategies	Vijay and colleagues' (2016) comparison of the costs of brief interventions for increasing physical activity levels
Umbrella review or overview	A review of the other reviews in a topic area. Searches are exhaustive and there is critical appraisal of located reviews	Sweet and Fortier's (2010) synthesis of meta-analysis and systematic reviews on the effect of health behaviour interventions on physical activity and diet

Source Adapted from Grant and Booth (2009) and Booth et al. (2016)

□ Table 1.2 presents examples of methods for synthesizing qualitative literature. Meta-ethnographies synthesis interpretative accounts of a phenomenon with reviewers typically translating concepts from one account into another, exploring contradictions among accounts and developing lines of argument. When undertaking a meta-study, reviewers examine primary studies' methods, data, and theories separately before each contributes to a meta-synthesis of the literature. In a meta-narrative, investigators explore the evolution of different narratives within a topic area's evidence base. A realist synthesis reviews the evidence for the theory underpinning an intervention.

□ Table 1.2   Examples of review methods suitable for synthesizing qualitative evidence

Review type and key reference	Description	Example
Meta-ethnography, Noblit and Hare (1988)	A review designed to synthesis interpretative accounts of phenomena. Typical synthesis methods include translating concepts from one account into another (*reciprocal translation analysis*), exploring contradictions among accounts (*refutational synthesis*), and developing a larger understanding of the phenomenon from accounts of its components (*Lines-of-argument synthesis*)	Soundy and colleagues (2012) meta-ethnography on the psychosocial processes involved in physical activity and mental illness
Meta-study, Paterson et al. (2001)	A multifaceted approach in which separate examinations of primary studies' methods, data, and theories each contribute to a meta-synthesis of the literature	Holt and colleagues' (2017) examination of positive youth development through sport
Meta-narrative, Greenhalgh et al. (2005)	An approach focused on identifying the evolution of different narratives within the evidence associated with an area of study	Timpka and colleagues (2015) meta-narrative of sports injury reporting practices in athletics
Realist synthesis, Pawson et al. (2004)	A method focused on synthesizing evidence attesting to the mid-level or programme theories underpinning interventions. The driving question is what works for whom, under what circumstances, in what ways, and how?	Harden and colleagues' (2015) examination on achieving success in group-based physical activity interventions

Researchers may wonder how many primary studies are needed to warrant doing a review, and there is no absolute answer. Given that systematic reviewing is a process, it is feasible to complete a well-conducted empty review in which no primary investigations are found. Empty reviews provide clear answers about the quality and quantity of existing evidence for a research question: there is none. Becoming aware of what we do not know is as useful as what we do know. The litmus test, however, is what contribution does the review make to the knowledge base? Sometimes, an empty review may draw attention to a phenomenon deserving consideration. For example, practitioners may start believing that a new intervention helps athletes enhance performance because of slick marketing and promotion. An empty review might highlight that they need to be more discerning in their professional judgement. There are more manuscripts vying for journal space than can be published, however. Empty reviews are likely to be published rarely. Nevertheless, it is an arbitrary decision regarding the number of studies needed and more does not always signal a contribution (Petticrew & Roberts, 2006). Multiple reviews on the same topic risk wasteful duplication of effort and resources (Ioannidis, 2016). In trendy research areas, reviewers enhance their case for publication by demonstrating how their projects plug a hole, provide new insights, or can support decision-making.

1

Systematic reviewers typically value transparent and methodical methods (Mallett, Hagen-Zanker, Slater, & Duvendack, 2012), but beyond these generally agreed benchmarks, people debate several beliefs about the genre. To illustrate, whereas Chandler et al.'s (2017) description states there is an attempt to include all evidence in a review, other methodologists argue that such a criterion is not always required (Brunton, Stansfield, Caird, & Thomas, 2017). It is desirable to include all available evidence in a meta-analysis to help increase the accuracy and precision of the estimated effect size (Borenstein, Hedges, Higgins, & Rothstein, 2009). In a meta-narrative, however, where the focus is on identifying lines of research within a body of knowledge, it may be acceptable to focus on seminal or influential documents rather than trying to synthesize all the literature (Greenhalgh et al., 2005).

Although opinions differ about many aspects in systematic reviewing, people agree on some ways by which these projects may be classified. One common classification involves aggregation versus configuration (Gough, Thomas, & Oliver, 2012; Voils, Sandelowski, Barroso, & Hasselblad, 2008). In aggregative reviews, investigators normally collect and assimilate evidence to describe and test pre-determined constructs and relationships. The evidence is aggregated, and often averaged, to allow theory testing to occur. Meta-analyses are usually aggregative, because they produce a weighted average from an array of numbers (e.g., mean differences and sample sizes) to reflect a summary effect size. Answers from aggregative reviews are most reliable when the studies underpinning analysis are homogeneous. The presence of heterogeneity or variation in the studies' characteristics likely introduces inaccuracy to aggregated findings. Males and females, for example, normally score drive for muscularity scales differently. Reviewers who combine male and female samples in calculating average drive for muscularity scores likely return a result that represents neither gender.

In a configural review, by contrast, evidence is interpreted and arranged in ways to generate a new understanding of the topic. The methods in ◻ Table 1.2 are examples of configural reviews. Studies do not have to be homogenous and variation may be favoured. Methods for reviewing qualitative investigations, for example, often focus on seeking novel ways to combine research to allow constructs to emerge with the aim being to develop, broaden, or deepen theory. The aggregative and configural distinction is not absolute. Meta-analyses, for instance, can help develop, as well as test, theory, and qualitative research may be aggregated if doing so answers the review question.

Chapter Case Example: Do the Olympic Games Increase Sport Participation?

In 2015, Weed and colleagues published a systematic review examining evidence that major sporting events, such as the Olympic Games, influence sports participation. Their review illustrates the typical structure and components of systematic reviews. If you have access to the *European Sport Management Quarterly*, then you can read the article (it appeared in volume 15, issue 2, pages 195–226). Alternatively, a pre-published version is available online at the Canterbury Christ Church University's and Brunel University's research archives. Reading this summary and Weed et al.'s report will assist you in understanding systematic reviews and will help you as you read the following chapters. You may find it easier to see how the information in each chapter fits within systematic review development, undertaking, and presentation.

Review questions

Weed and colleagues set out to answer two explicit questions (p. 202): *"what evidence exists that previous Olympic games, sport events or sport franchises have impacted upon sport participation?"* and *"by what processes has sport participation been leveraged from previous Olympic Games, sport events or sport franchises?"* The review introduction explains why the questions are relevant, will advance knowledge, and provide useful information for decision-making support. Systematic reviews, particularly those drawing on a sizeable knowledgebase, involve significant labour and resources. Careful reviewers consider whether or not the likely output is worth them foregoing the other activities they might undertake, such as conducting primary research, writing grant applications, or watching The Simpsons.

Method

Weed et al. provide a detailed description of the literature search in which they discuss their pilot work to develop the electronic search strategy and keywords. They also present details of alternative sources

of information, such as relevant organizations, unindexed archives, and the reference lists of located literature. A flow chart is presented summarizing the search, including the number of initial documents located (1778) through to the identification on the final 21 studies that were reviewed. Additional details describe the basis on which articles were excluded or included, so readers can assess the adequacy of the search and selection of the final studies.

The authors also detail how they assessed the quality of the included literature. Rather than using a standardized quality assessment tool, they created one (presented in their appendix) tailored to their needs. Weed et al. justified the items they included on their critical appraisal form, which focused on relevance, quality, and ethics. A table presents the results of the quality appraisal for each of the included studies to allow readers to discern trends across the body of literature.

The data analysis procedure is presented at the start of the results (in many reviews this is located in the method section), and involved a semi-inductive thematic analysis. The product was a critical narrative synthesis, which allowed the authors to both summarize the knowledge contained in the evidence and highlight weaknesses in the reviewed research.

One reason why I selected Weed et al.'s work for this chapter was because it illustrates how systematic reviews can involve a narrative examination integrating both qualitative and quantitative evidence.

Results

In line with the semi-inductive thematic analysis, the results were presented within two pre-determined higher order themes derived from the research questions. The approach ensured the authors provided clear answers to their review questions. They focused on the sport participation outcomes that might result from major sporting events, and the processes that might help leverage those effects. The authors concluded that leveraging a demonstration effect, whereby elite events and athletes inspire people to engage in sport, in the led up to the Olympic Games may increase participation frequency and potentially re-engage lapsed individuals. Relying on an inherent demonstration effect, however, to attract new individuals to start playing sport is unlikely to be successful.

Discussion

The authors discuss how their findings contribute to the literature. They also position the findings in the real world by evaluating the legacy claims of the 2012 London Olympics. A second reason why I presented Weed et al. (2015) is

1

because it is an example of the contribution systematic reviews may make to help real-world decision-making. A justification for holding major sporting events is the belief that such showpieces will inspire people to become active in sport. Rather than seeing the answer to the question as dichotomous, Weed et al. (2015) conclude that:

If the primary justification for hosting an Olympic Games is the potential impact on sport participation, the Games are a bad investment. However, the Games can have specific impacts on sport participation frequency and re-engagement, and if these are desirable for host societies, are properly leveraged by hosts, and are one among a number of reasons for hosting the Games, then the Games may be a justifiable investment in sport participation terms.

Weed et al. provides a careful and balanced assessment of the evidence that policymakers, practitioners, and individuals can consider when making decisions about whether or not to bid for major sporting events. Such decisions are unlikely to be based solely on one or even several systematic reviews. These decisions are political exercises and involve debate over personal and collective values, beliefs, and interests. Systematic reviews of evidence, however, can inform those decisions and help people clarify where they stand on specific issues. Systematic reviews are one of a number of information sources that can help societies determine the ways they wish to organize and run themselves.

Summary

The big bang theory is a cosmological model describing how the universe started small but expanded to become momentous. The model could be applied to research in sport, exercise, and physical activity. The literature base has become large, has fragmented greatly, and appears to be expanding at an accelerating rate. Traditionally, experts might have been able to keep abreast of research in their topic areas with relative ease and little effort, but this is no longer possible for most areas, and especially those that have relevance for modern societies' most pressing needs and challenges. The systematic review process represents a way for authors to generate an understanding of current knowledge and the quality of the under-pinning evidence. Such an approach allows greater precision in understanding and minimizing potential biases in knowledge advancement. The results from these projects can contribute to decision-making. The systematic review process can help us (a) understand what is *it* that we know, (b) appreciate the basis on which we know *it*, and (c) decide what we are going to do about *it*.

❓ Learning Exercises

1. Find a traditional "black box" review and a systematic synthesis from within your area of interest or specialty, if possible dealing with a similar topic.
   − To what degree is each of them transparent, rigorous, and reproducible?

— How confident are you in their findings? That is, did the authors evaluate the quality of the included literature (and do something with this information) and did they undertake a process that minimized undue bias?
— How well do you believe each review could provide knowledge and decision-making support?

2. Find a systematic review within your area and evaluate it in light of the PRISMA checklist. The PRISMA (Preferred Reporting Items for Systematic Reviews and Meta-Analyses) checklist is set of items aimed at helping authors ensure transparent and complete reporting of systematic reviews and meta-analyses. Although generated for medical and health research, and designed for systematic reviews of RCTs, it can be used for reporting reviews of other types of research. The PRISMA checklist may be downloaded from the PRISMA website (▶ http://www.prisma-statement.org/) or it can be found in Moher, Liberati, Tetzlaff, Altman, and The Prisma Group (2009). Based on your assessment, did you identify any weaknesses in the review? Did your perceptions about the review change after applying the PRISMA checklist?

3. If you have a topic in which you are interested, locate 2–3 book chapters, systematic reviews, or traditional black box reviews to help you develop an overview of what is known about the area. Generate some ideas out of which you might be able to form a systematic review question. Reflect on the following to help you identify possibilities: are there any gaps in the evidence that you think are important to address? What specific populations, activities, and outcomes do you think are important to find out about? You will use these ideas to create a review protocol discussed in the next chapter.

References

Booth, A., Sutton, A., & Papaioannou, D. (2016). *Systematic approaches to a successful literature review* (2nd ed.). Thousand Oaks, CA: Sage.

Borenstein, M., Hedges, L. V., Higgins, J. P. T., & Rothstein, H. R. (2009). *Introduction to meta-analysis*. Chichester, UK: Wiley.

Brunton, G., Stansfield, C., Caird, J., & Thomas, J. (2017). Finding relevant studies. In D. Gough, S. Oliver, & J. Thomas (Eds.), *An introduction to systematic reviews* (2nd ed., pp. 93–122). Thousand Oaks, CA: Sage.

Chalmers, I., Hedges, L. V., & Cooper, H. (2002). A brief history of research synthesis. *Evaluation and the Health Professions, 25*, 12–37. ▶ https://doi.org/10.1177/0163278702025001003.

Chandler, J., Higgins, J. P. T., Deeks, J. J., Davenport, C., & Clarke, M. J. (2017). Introduction. In J. P. T. Higgins, R. Churchill, J. Chandler, & M. S. Cumpston (Eds.), *Cochrane handbook for systematic reviews of interventions (version 5.2.0)*. Retrieved from ▶ www.training.cochrane.org/handbook.

Cochrane, A. L. (1972). *Effectiveness and efficiency: Random reflections on health services*. London, UK: Nuffield Provincial Hospitals Trust.

Cochrane, A. L. (1979). 1931–1971: A critical review with particular reference to the medical profession. In G. Teeling-Smith & N. Wells (Eds.), *Medicines for the year 2000* (pp. 2–12). London, UK: Office for Health Economics.

Edwards, S., & Launder, C. (2000). Investigating muscularity concerns in male body image: Development of the Swansea Muscularity Attitudes Questionnaire. *International Journal of Eating Disorders, 28*, 120–124. ▶ https://doi.org/10.1002/(SICI)1098-108X(200007)28:1<120::AID-EAT15>3.0.CO;2-H.

Gough, D., Oliver, S., & Thomas, J. (2017). Introducing systematic reviews. In D. Gough, S. Oliver, & J. Thomas (Eds.), *An introduction to systematic reviews* (2nd ed., pp. 1–17). Thousand Oaks, CA: Sage.

Gough, D., Thomas, J., & Oliver, S. (2012). Clarifying differences between review designs and methods. *Systematic Reviews, 1,* 1–9. ► https://doi.org/10.1186/2046-4053-1-28.

Grant, M. J., & Booth, A. (2009). A typology of reviews: An analysis of 14 review types and associated methodologies. *Health Information & Libraries Journal, 26,* 91–108. ► https://doi.org/10.1111/j.1471-1842.2009.00848.x.

Greenhalgh, T., Robert, G., Macfarlane, F., Bate, P., Kyriakidou, O., & Peacock, R. (2005). Storylines of research in diffusion of innovation: A meta-narrative approach to systematic review. *Social Science and Medicine, 61,* 417–430. ► https://doi.org/10.1016/j.socscimed.2004.12.001.

Hammersley, M. (2006). Systematic or unsystematic, is that the question? Some reflections on the science, art, and politics of reviewing research evidence. In A. Killoran, C. Swann, & M. P. Kelly (Eds.), *Public health evidence: Tackling health inequalities* (pp. 239–250). Oxford, UK: Oxford University Press.

Harden, S. M., McEwan, D., Sylvester, B. D., Kaulius, M., Ruissen, G., Burke, S. M., Estabrooks, P. A., & Beauchamp, M. R. (2015). Understanding for whom, under what conditions, and how group-based physical activity interventions are successful: A realist review. *BMC Public Health, 15,* article 958. ► https://doi.org/10.1186/s12889-015-2270-8.

Holt, N. L., Neely, K. C., Slater, L. G., Camiré, M., Côté, J., Fraser-Thomas, J., MacDonald, D., Strachan, L., & Tamminen, K. A. (2017). A grounded theory of positive youth development through sport based on results from a qualitative meta-study. *International Review of Sport and Exercise Psychology, 10,* 1–49. ► https://doi.org/10.1080/1750984X.2016.1180704.

Langer, L. (2015). Sport for development—A systematic map of evidence from Africa. *South African Review of Sociology, 46,* 66–86. ► https://doi.org/10.1080/21528586.2014.989665.

Ioannidis, J. P. A. (2016). The mass production of redundant, misleading, and conflicted systematic reviews and meta-analyses. *The Milbank Quarterly, 94,* 485–514. ► https://doi.org/10.1111/1468-0009.12210.

Macnamara, B. N., Moreau, D., & Hambrick, D. Z. (2016). The relationship between deliberate practice and performance in sports: A meta-analysis. *Perspectives on Psychological Science, 11,* 333–350. ► https://doi.org/10.1177/1745691616635591.

Mallett, R., Hagen-Zanker, J., Slater, R., & Duvendack, M. (2012). The benefits and challenges of using systematic reviews in international development research. *Journal of Development Effectiveness, 4,* 445–455. ► https://doi.org/10.1080/19439342.2012.711342.

Martin, A., Booth, J. N., Laird, Y., Sproule, J., Reilly, J. J., & Saunders, D. H. (2018). Physical activity, diet and other behavioural interventions for improving cognition and school achievement in children and adolescents with obesity or overweight. *Cochrane Database of Systematic Reviews.* Retrieved from ► www.cochranelibrary.com. ► https://doi.org/10.1002/14651858.CD009728.pub3.

McCreary, D. R., & Sasse, D. K. (2000). An exploration of the drive for muscularity in adolescent boys and girls. *Journal of American College Health, 48,* 297–304. ► https://doi.org/10.1080/07448480009596271.

Moher, D., Liberati, A., Tetzlaff, J., Altman, D. G., & The Prisma Group. (2009). Preferred reporting items for systematic reviews and meta-analyses: The PRISMA statement. *PLoS Medicine, 6,* e1000097. ► https://doi.org/10.1371/journal.pmed.1000097.

Mulrow, C. D. (1987). The medical review article: State of the science. *Annals of Internal Medicine, 106,* 485–488. ► https://doi.org/10.7326/0003-4819-106-3-485.

NICE. (2014). *Physical activity: Exercise referral schemes.* London, UK: Author.

Noblit, G. W., & Hare, R. D. (1988). *Meta-ethnography: Synthesizing qualitative studies.* Thousand Oaks, CA: Sage.

Oxman, A. D., & Guyatt, G. H. (1993). The science of reviewing research. *Annals of the New York Academy of Sciences, 703,* 125–134. ► https://doi.org/10.1111/j.1749-6632.1993.tb26342.x.

Page, M. J., Shamseer, L., Altman, D. G., Tetzlaff, J., Sampson, M., Tricco, A. C., … Moher, D. (2016). Epidemiology and reporting characteristics of systematic reviews of biomedical research: A cross-sectional study. *PLoS Medicine, 13,* e1002028. ► https://doi.org/10.1371/journal.pmed.1002028.

Paterson, B. L., Thorne, S. E., Canam, C., & Jillings, C. (2001). *Meta-study of qualitative health research: A practical guide to meta-analysis and meta-synthesis*. Thousand Oaks, CA: Sage.

Pawson, R., Greenhalgh, T., Harvey, G., & Walshe, K. (2004). *Realist synthesis: An introduction*. Manchester, UK: Economic and Social Research Council.

Petticrew, M. (2001). Systematic reviews from astronomy to zoology: Myths and misconceptions. *British Medical Journal, 322*, 98–101. ▶ https://doi.org/10.1136/bmj.322.7278.98.

Petticrew, M., & Roberts, H. (2006). *Systematic reviews in the social sciences: A practical guide*. Malden, MA: Blackwell.

Pope, C., Mays, N., & Popay, J. (2007). *Synthesising qualitative and quantitative health evidence: A guide to methods*. Maidenhead, UK: Open University Press.

Sacks, H. S., Berrier, J., Reitman, D., Ancona-Berk, V. A., & Chalmers, T. C. (1987). Meta-analyses of randomized controlled trials. *New England Journal of Medicine, 316*, 450–455. ▶ https://doi.org/10.1056/NEJM198702193160806.

Soundy, A., Kingstone, T., & Coffee, P. (2012). Understanding the psychosocial processes of physical activity for individuals with severe mental illness: A meta-ethnography. In L. L'Abate (Ed.), *Mental illnesses—Evaluation, treatments and implications* (pp. 3–20). Rijeka, Croatia: InTech.

Stork, M. J., Banfield, L. E., Gibala, M. J., & Martin Ginis, K. A. (2017). A scoping review of the psychological responses to interval exercise: Is interval exercise a viable alternative to traditional exercise? *Health Psychology Review, 11*, 324–344. ▶ https://doi.org/10.1080/17437199.2017.1326011.

Sweet, S. N., & Fortier, M. S. (2010). Improving physical activity and dietary behaviours with single or multiple health behaviour interventions? A synthesis of meta-analyses and reviews. *International Journal of Environmental Research and Public Health, 7*, 1720–1743. ▶ https://doi.org/10.3390/ijerph7041720.

Timpka, T., Jacobsson, J., Ekberg, J., Finch, C. F., Bichenbach, J., Edouard, P., Bargoria, V., Branco, P., & Alonso, J. M. (2015). Meta-narrative analysis of sports injury reporting practices based on the Injury Definitions Concept Framework (IDCF): A review of consensus statements and epidemiological studies in athletics (track and field). *Journal of Science and Medicine in Sport, 18*, 643–650. ▶ https://doi.org/10.1016/j.jsams.2014.11.393.

Tod, D., & Eubank, M. (2017). Conducting a systematic review: Demystification for trainees in sport and exercise psychology. *Sport and Exercise Psychology Review, 13*(1), 65–72.

Vijay, G. C., Wilson, E. C. F., Suhrcke, M., Hardeman, W., & Sutton, S. (2016). Are brief interventions to increase physical activity cost-effective? A systematic review. *British Journal of Sports Medicine, 50*, 408–417. ▶ https://doi.org/10.1136/bjsports-2015-094655.

Voils, C. I., Sandelowski, M., Barroso, J., & Hasselblad, V. (2008). Making sense of qualitative and quantitative findings in mixed research synthesis studies. *Field Methods, 20*, 3–25. ▶ https://doi.org/10.1177/1525822X07307463.

Ware, M., & Mabe, M. (2015). *The STM report: An overview of scientific and scholarly journal publishing*. The Hague, The Netherlands: International Association of Scientific, Technical, and Medical Publishers.

Weed, M., Coren, E., Fiore, J., Wellard, I., Chatziefstathiou, D., Mansfield, L., & Dowse, S. (2015). The Olympic Games and raising sport participation: A systematic review of evidence and an interrogation of policy for a demonstration effect. *European Sport Management Quarterly, 15*, 195–226. ▶ https://doi.org/10.1080/16184742.2014.998695.

Planning a Review

D. Tod, *Conducting Systematic Reviews in Sport, Exercise, and Physical Activity*,
https://doi.org/10.1007/978-3-030-12263-8_2

2

Learning Objectives

After reading this chapter, you should be able to:
- Describe features involved in the systematic review process.
- Discuss benefits of developing and registering review protocols.
- Write a review protocol.
- Apply project management principles to systematic reviewing.
- Audit your systematic review competencies.

Introduction

I suggested in ▶ Chapter 1 that sport, exercise, and physical activity-related systematic reviews somewhat echoed primary research, but the samples included research papers (or other types of evidence) instead of humans. The analogy helps illuminate the review process. Both reviews and primary research are examples of creative problem-solving. Researchers identify a problem (pose a question), determine possible solutions (create a method), implement favoured options (collect data), assess consequences (data analysis), and determine implications (data interpretation). One attraction of (and justification for) conducting research or reviews is the opportunity to solve problems or offer solutions that improve society and people's lives. For both research and problem solving, optimal results are more likely if people work towards a goal in logical ways, rather than wander around without a plan. Similarly, to complete influential systematic reviews, it is helpful to have a guiding map. In this chapter, I will focus on the systematic review map and the first major milestone: a protocol.

Systematic Review Elements: The 4Cs

The 4Cs of systematic reviews are illustrated in ◘ Fig. 2.1, and include *conceptualizing, constructing, conducting,* and *communicating* projects, echoing the primary research process (Arthur & Hancock, 2009). Typically, authors suggest systematic reviews should follow a series of discrete steps in a linear manner. Some projects may proceed in such a way, including aggregative reviews or those answering narrow specific questions, drawing on a clearly identified research base, and using accepted analysis techniques. As implied in ◘ Fig. 2.1, however, reviews may also occur in a cyclical fashion, with authors switching back and forth across activities. Furthermore, for some types of reviews iteration is built into the procedures, such as those designed for synthesizing qualitative research, or for situations where it is not possible to determine methods prior to starting, for example, projects focussed on theory development (Pawson, Greenhalgh, Harvey, & Walshe, 2004). Rather than dictating a linear multi-staged approach, it is more accurate to suggest there are various elements needing consideration (Pope, Mays, & Popay, 2007). The journey starts with conceptualization, but the final path varies according to the needs of the project.

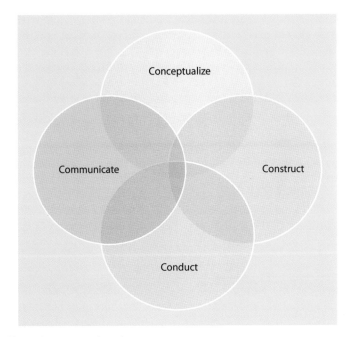

◘ Fig. 2.1 Phases in a systematic review

Conceptualize the review   When conceptualizing reviews, researchers refine, as much as possible, the guiding questions. They also scope the literature to establish the feasibility of answering those questions and invite feedback from stakeholders. A third task is to justify the review in terms of knowledge or decision making support.

Construct the method   The major goal during construction is to propose methods that flow from the questions. Coherency between the questions and methods ensures that suitable answers are produced. Although many factors influence a review's purpose, such as stakeholders, resources, and authors themselves, the question needs to be a major guiding force when designing the method. If reviewers do not ensure question-method coherency, they limit their ability to provide meaningful answers or produce reports that contribute to knowledge or help people make decisions. For example, reviewers wishing to estimate the strength of the relationship between two variables will adopt meta-analytic methods, rather than qualitative approaches. Meta-analyses, however, are less helpful in answering questions focused on understanding how people interpret and make sense of their experiences; a job better suited to methods that synthesis qualitative work.

Activities undertaken during method construction include identifying:
- The type of research to be reviewed.
- The search strategies and keywords that will locate evidence.
- The data extraction and critical appraisal tools.
- The makeup of the research team to ensure necessary competencies are available.
- The logistical and ethical considerations needing to be addressed.

2

Pilot work may be undertaken to evaluate possible review methods (Long, 2014). Reviewers, often, do not need to start from ground zero, but can draw on established methods, such as those presented in ▶ Chapter 1. A major milestone in the construction phase is a review protocol allowing for feedback from colleagues and stakeholders.

Conduct the review   Systematic reviews take time and energy. Some students I have supervised (and colleagues I have collaborated with) experience doubt when undertaking reviews, because they are uncertain if they will do a fine job. They may also be overwhelmed when they realize the amount of work often involved. Those folks with perfectionist tendencies sometimes want assurances that their methods will generate results or the journey will be trouble-free. Unlike death and taxes, however, systematic reviews are probabilistic undertakings and desired results are not guaranteed. Nonetheless, the more time people spend constructing, piloting, and seeking feedback on their methods, the better their chances of answering their questions.

Communicate the findings   As suggested in ▶ Chapter 1, systematic reviews are seldom written for the author's pleasure, but for audiences who include fellow researchers, practitioners, and decision makers. Authors who consider their audiences' expectations and needs increase the likelihood their reviews will be well-received and influential. For example, if planning a review on preventing falls in elderly individuals, investigators might ask exercise professionals or older individuals what questions would be worth posing and how answers can be best disseminated.

Most reviews are published in a written format, and authors who consider the quality of their writing and the coherency of the content will increase the influence of their work. Well-written reviews allow readers to identify the golden threads and take-home messages. Systematic reviews are scientific reports and the prose needs to conform to social expectations associated with technical writing (Pinker, 2015). A rigorous systematic review that answers a meaningful question, and has a clear message, will be an engaging read for interested parties.

Systematic reviews provide authors opportunities to discuss applied implications and future research avenues. In both cases, specific suggestions that are clearly linked to the review's results provide the greatest punch. Statements, for example, such as "more research is needed" are vague and unhelpful. Readers can justifiably expect authors who have reviewed the evidence to either provide concrete and specific suggestions or explain why they cannot forward any recommendations (e.g., lack of suitable evidence). Applied implications may not be feasible or needed, but if authors are going to provide them, then seeking feedback from potential audiences helps ensure the usefulness of the recommendations.

Various reporting standards exist to facilitate the production of complete clear reports, such as the PRISMA checklist introduced in ▶ Chapter 1. The PRISMA checklist is suitable for syntheses of experimental research. Authors can, however, select from other standards if reviewing different research designs, such as the Meta-analysis Of Observational Studies in Epidemiology (MOOSE) guidelines when meta-analysing survey research (Stroup et al., 2000). The Enhancing Transparency in Reporting the synthesis of Qualitative research (ENTREQ) checklist is tailored towards reviews of qualitative work (Tong, Flemming, McInnes, Oliver, & Craig, 2012). The RAMESES project (▶ http://www.ramesesproject.org) has produced reporting standards for realist syntheses and meta-narrative reviews.

Benefits of Developing and Registering Review Protocols

Developing a protocol has several benefits and is a useful milestone when constructing review methods (Moher et al., 2015; Shamseer et al., 2015). For example, through planning and documenting the protocol, reviewers develop a description of the end result, giving them a clear sense of direction. When multiple people are involved, protocols ensure the team members have a shared understanding of their goals and how each person contributes to the outputs. Protocols enhance decision making consistency, because authors determine their rulebook prior to conducting the project. A protocol assists accountability, because it provides a basis against which the review can be judged (Moher et al., 2015). Developing a protocol may involve piloting review methods and seeking feedback from others, including researchers, librarians, methodology experts, and members of intended audiences, to ensure the design is feasible and likely to return a useful product. Such feedback may assist students or inexperienced reviewers who need guidance from supervisors. Written protocols in such instances reduce misunderstandings that arise in spoken communication.

Once reviewers have written their protocols, they may consider registering them with relevant organizations, such as PROSPERO (▶ https://www.crd.york.ac.uk/prospero/). PROSPERO is a global database of prospectively registered systematic reviews focused on at least one health-related outcome. The reviews come from various fields, including health and social care, welfare, public health, education, crime, justice, and international development. Other examples of organizations where reviews can be registered are the Cochrane Collaboration, the Campbell Collaboration, the Joanna Briggs Institute, and the Best Evidence Medical Education collaboration.

Some journals and organizations stipulate that registration is a requirement for purposes such as funding or publication. The PRISMA website, for example, keeps a list of organizations and journals that endorse the PRISMA standards of reporting. A number of these journals are outlets where researchers in sport, exercise, and physical activity may wish to submit their reviews, such as *BMC Public Health, Lancet,* and the *Journal of Health Psychology.*

Several benefits exist for registering protocols (Booth, Sutton, & Papaioannou, 2016; Mallett, Hagen-Zanker, Slater, & Duvendack, 2012). It helps review teams stake their claim over a topic and lets interested parties know of their intentions. Advertising one's objectives may bring people together and help reviewers make contact with other experts who have relevant skills and resources. Such networking may lead to better outputs. For the scientific community and wider society, registration assists with the identification of reporting bias, or selective outcome reporting, whereby authors make ad hoc decisions about what results to include from primary studies after they have begun their projects (Page, McKenzie, & Forbes, 2013; Tricco et al., 2016). For example, authors may not include findings they had intended to report, because they were non-significant or conflicted with theory. Alternatively, they may include outcomes they had not intended on reporting, but for which they found significant results. Evidence indicates that these changes are seldom acknowledged, documented, or justified (Tricco et al., 2016). Publically available protocols allow authors' work to be judged against their initial intentions to assist in identifying biased reporting.

Another benefit is the reduction of duplicated effort (Moher et al., 2015). A balance needs to be struck, however, because although it is wasteful to use limited resources to duplicate systematic reviews unnecessarily, evidence reveals authors examining the same or similar topics produce different results (Jadad, Cook, & Browman, 1997). Systematic review findings may conflict because (a) of variation in methods employed, (b) researchers used incorrect or outdated techniques, or (c) investigators did not undertake the process rigorously (Ioannidis, 2016). Replication has a role in science, although authors need to justify the duplication.

A Possible Protocol Structure

To illustrate the content that can be included in a protocol and a possible structure, ◧ Table 2.1 lists the content required in a PRISMA protocol (PRISMA-P, Moher et al., 2015). The first few items (1–3) focus on administrative details to help people identify the project, such as title, contributors, registration database and number, and correspondence details. The amendments section (item 4) allows investigators to update protocols and document any changes they have made since registering their projects. Sometimes reviewers need to adjust protocols after the project has begun, rather than sticking dogmatically to methods they believe to be no longer suitable. Documenting and justifying changes helps to reduce suspicions about biased reporting if the final report is different from the initial protocol. Returning to the protocol in ◧ Table 2.1, details about support (item 5) help determine conflicts of interest.

The protocol introduction serves a similar purpose to its counterpart in primary research: authors justify their projects. Providing a rationale (item 6) helps convince readers the review is worth doing. The PRISMA-P then presents the review purpose (item 7). The PICO acronym is one of several frameworks that help authors define their driving questions and stands for Population, Intervention, Comparison, and Outcome (see ▶ Chapter 3). An example question might be:

- In elderly females (*Population*)
- What effect does a community walking programme (*Intervention*)
- Compared with a book club (*Comparison*)
- Have on their sense of independence, autonomy, and relatedness (*Outcomes*)?

The PICO framework signals implicitly that the PRISMA-P is tailored towards reviews of experimental work or randomized controlled trials (Shamseer et al., 2015), and may need modification if authors focus on non-intervention research.

The methods section (items 8–17) is where reviewers record how they are going to identify relevant literature, extract information from selected studies, assess risk of bias, and process data to obtain answers to the review questions. Ideally, the level

◻ Table 2.1 Content of a PRISMA-P protocol (Moher et al., 2015)

Information	Item	Description (item number)
Administrative information		
Title	1a	Identify the document as a systematic review protocol
	1b	Explain if it for an update of a previous project
Registration	2	If relevant, indicate registration number and registry
Authors	3a	Contact details including name, institutional affiliation, and e-mail address of all protocol authors. Also include corresponding author's physical mailing address
	3b	Present each authors' contributions and the review guarantor
Amendments	4	Identify if the protocol includes amendments from a previously completed or published protocol, along with the changes. Otherwise outline a plan for documenting changes
Support	5a	Indicate sources of financial or other support for the review
	5b	Provide names of sponsors or funders
	5c	Detail the roles of funders, sponsors, and/or institutions in developing the protocol
Introduction		
Rationale	6	Describe the rationale for the review in the context of what is already known
Objectives	7	Outline an explicit statement of the review questions with reference to participants, interventions, comparators, and outcomes (PICO)
Methods		
Eligibility criteria	8	Specify study characteristics, such as PICO, design, setting, timeframe, and report characteristics to be used as eligibility criteria for the review (e.g., years considered, language, publication status)
Information sources	9	Describe all intended information sources, including electronic databases, contact with study authors, trial registers, or other grey literature sources, with planned dates of coverage
Search strategy	10	Present a draft of at least one electronic database search strategy sufficiently that it could be repeated, including planned limits
Study records	11a	Describe mechanisms for managing records and data
	11b	State processes for selecting studies (e.g., two independent reviewers) throughout each review phase
	11c	Describe methods for extracting data from reports (e.g., piloting forms, done independently, in duplicate), and any processes for obtaining and confirming data from investigators
Data items	12	List and define variables for which data will be sought, any preplanned data assumptions and simplifications

(continued)

2

⊠ Table 2.1 (continued)

Information	Item	Description (item number)
Outcomes and prioritization	13	List and define all outcomes for which data will be sought, including prioritization of main and additional outcomes, with rationale
Risk of bias in individual studies	14	Describe anticipated methods for assessing individual study risk of bias, including whether this will be done at the outcome level, study level, or both. Indicate how this information will be used in data synthesis
Data synthesis	15a	Describe criteria under which data will be synthesized quantitatively
	15b	If data are appropriate for quantitative synthesis, describe planned summary measures, methods of handling data, and methods of combining data from studies, including any planned exploration of consistency (e.g., I^2, Kendall's tau)
	15c	Describe proposed additional analyses (e.g., sensitivity or subgroup analyses, meta-regression)
	15d	If quantitative synthesis is inappropriate, describe the type of summary planned
Meta-biases	16	Specify planned meta-biases assessment (e.g., publication bias, selective reporting)
Confidence in cumulative evidence	17	Describe how the strength of the evidence will be assessed (e.g., GRADE)

of detail provided in a protocol is sufficient to allow readers to replicate the study. As might be expected given that PRISMA-P is directed towards randomized controlled trials, the items about data analysis are focused on meta-analysis (items 15–16). Item 15d, however, allows for other types of analysis, such as qualitative approaches.

Despite its leanings towards the meta-analysis of randomized controlled trials, PRISMA-P may be modified for other types of reviews and could be used in a wide variety of contexts. For example, supervisors might ask students to use PRISMA-P to develop a protocol for their studies. These protocols can be shared within and outside of the supervision team for feedback purposes. Although the PRISMA-P is useful, other protocol templates exist, including the PROSPERO version illustrated in the chapter case example below.

Applying Project Management Principles to the Review Process

Undertaking a review is an exercise in project management, or the implementation of resources, personnel, processes, knowledge, skills, and experience to achieve a discrete endeavour's objectives (Mesly, 2017). Insights from project management can help individuals to complete their research syntheses efficiently and effectively. Numerous Ps are involved in project management, but five worthy of contemplation for reviewers are *Product, Plan, People, Process,* and *Power.*

Product   Investigators who understand the shape that their final reviews will take can make decisions about how they can reach the project's desired destination. They can include the intended audience in outlining the final product, such as asking stakeholders about the questions they want answered or how the findings can be presented. Other considerations include the identifying methods that will provide coherent answers to the questions.

Plan   Planning involves team members developing a road map that will guide their activities. Once people get immersed in their data search, extraction, analysis, and synthesis, they realize how messy systematic reviews can become and how tempting it is to explore unintended topics. The project's road map helps keep people on course. Such plans, however, also need to be flexible. Sometimes it is worth exploring unintended areas, but a plan will help people make informed decisions about whether they have the scope and time to wander off the highway to explore a byway. GANTT charts are one way to plan systematic reviews and record what activities will be undertaken, in what order, by whom, and by which dates. GANTT charts are visual descriptions of deliverable milestones, such as search completion, data analysis, and delivery of the final report.

People   Various skills, knowledge, and competencies are needed to complete reviews. Regarding knowledge, for example, it is helpful to have people who understand the content area being reviewed and those who understand the review process. Given the labour specialization involved in science, it is typically unusual for people to have knowledge in both domains. The assembly of competency-rich teams contributes to successful completion. Along with people's skills, knowledge, and competencies, it is worth considering how individuals get on with each other. People come with their motivations, personalities, tendencies, etc., and it is frustrating when projects stall because individuals fall out with each other.

Process   Whereas the plan is the roadmap outlining the systematic review journey, process refers to the mechanisms by which the vehicle will travel. Useful questions include how will people apply their knowledge, skills, and competencies to achieve project milestones? What resources will people need to complete their tasks?

Power   When conducting systematic reviews, power refers to the ability to influence the activities that occur. Often, systematic review teams in sport, exercise, and physical activity are small and power may be distributed equally. In larger teams, especially those undertaking funded projects that have many stakeholders, consideration of people's roles and authority may help avoid difficulties and provide ways to resolve differences among group members.

2

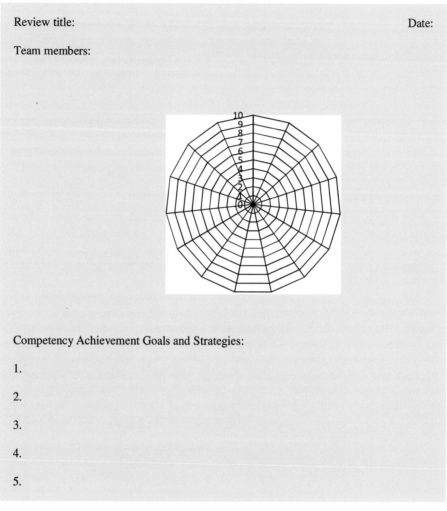

Review title: Date:

Team members:

Competency Achievement Goals and Strategies:

1.

2.

3.

4.

5.

◻ Fig. 2.2   A competency profiling worksheet

Profiling Your Systematic Review Competencies

Profiling helps individuals ascertain those relevant competencies they possess and those they are missing. Reflecting on one's competencies can bolster confidence or elicit attempts to ensure missing knowledge and skills are found. Profiling involves three stages, and ◻ Fig. 2.2 can help individuals undertake a profiling exercise:
1. Listing knowledge and skills needed to complete reviews.
2. Evaluating which competencies people have and which are missing.
3. Developing strategies to address deficits.

Stage 1: Identifying required competencies Profiling starts by generating a list of required skills and knowledge. Sometimes seeking input from others, such as librarians, experienced reviewers, and content experts, helps flesh out the list. Reading high quality reviews, and describing intended outputs, can stimulate additional ideas. For example, if the intended review will employ meta-narrative techniques, then having a person with literary criticism skills in the team will help increase the quality of data analysis and synthesis. ◘ Figure 2.2 has room for 15 competencies and stage 1 often results in a larger number of items. In these instances, it may be prudent to prioritize the list.

Stage 2: Rate the team's competence levels in these items ◘ Figure 2.2 allows individuals to rate themselves on a scale from 0 (not competent) to 10 (sufficiently competent). Although assessment is often subjective, drawing on concrete examples, where possible, helps improve the usefulness of profiling. For instance, if team members believe they are competent to apply meta-narrative methods, they can be asked to explain how they know they are capable or how they would apply the techniques to the project under question. Profiling is not an exact science, but a means to help teams work together to develop a common understanding of needed competences.

Stage 3: Address knowledge and skill deficits One outcome of stage 2 is a shared picture of a team's competencies and limitations. Having identified potential deficits, members can discuss strategies for fulling competency gaps and add these to ◘ Fig. 2.2. For example, members may realize that their literature search strategies are suited to a particular approach, and this may not be optimal for the new project. The team might schedule a training session with a librarian or invite the person to join the squad.

Chapter Case Example: Preventing Misuse of Muscle Enhancement Drugs

Bates et al. (in press) published a review on interventions to prevent the misuse of muscle enhancement drugs. They registered their protocol on PROSPERO (► http://www.crd.york.ac.uk/PROSPERO/display_record.php?ID=CRD42016051204). The document is free and you may find it helpful to have it next to you as I comment on its strengths and limitations. The protocol is a useful example to examine. First, many researchers in sport, exercise, and physical activity conduct systematic reviews involving health-related outcomes, and these projects would be eligible for PROSPERO registration. Second, PROSPERO protocols vary from the PRISMA-P checklist. Comparing the two types may help clarify the key information to include in protocols.

The initial section of Bates et al.'s protocol presents citation details, such as the title, registration number, and contributing authors, to help readers find the protocol in the PROSPERO database. In the next section, the four driving review questions are presented and broadly focus on (a) describing the characteristics and effectiveness of interventions and (b) exploring their theoretical basis. Unlike the PRISMA-P, the PROSPERO template did not require Bates et al. to provide a rationale for the review. Providing a rationale for a project, however, helps justify

2

the time and resources involved.

Following on, the protocol's search strategy is presented, beginning with a list of the electronic databases and keywords the authors aimed to use. The protocol also indicates how hand searching will be conducted and how grey literature will be located. After detailing the search strategy, the following details related to primary study eligibility are presented: (a) type of study, (b) condition or domain being examined, (c) population, (d) intervention/exposure, (e) control/comparison, (f) context, and (g) primary and secondary outcomes. One helpful feature of Bates et al.'s protocol is their justification of the search strategy and inclusion/exclusion criteria. For example, they excluded interventions focused on professional athletes, because of limited applicability to the general population. A survey of PROSPERO protocols suggests they can be descriptive, and readers may not always understand why reviewers have constructed their methods as presented. In other situations where individuals write review protocols, asking them to provide justifications for search strategies, inclusion/exclusion criteria, and any other method activities can have benefits. Asking students, for instance, to justify their methods allows them to demonstrate their understanding of

the process. As another example, providing justification helps authors reassure funders and other stakeholders that the project is feasible and will return desired outputs.

In the protocol's next section, Bates et al. describe the data extraction and management processes, including the specific information to be collected. A strong feature is reference to procedures to assess and monitor the accuracy and completeness of data extraction; specifically, an independent random review of 10% of the papers. Another positive aspect of the protocol is the explanation of how the authors will assess the theoretical basis of interventions. In primary research, investigators do not always make the theoretical basis of their interventions clear, even when they argue they have been theory-driven, and Bates et al. discussed how they would handle these studies.

The authors then explain how they will assess primary research risk of bias, indicating they will not exclude studies on the basis of quality. Quality assessment is an area where there exists great diversity of practice (as explained in ▶ Chapter 8). Some reviewers exclude studies identified as poor to ensure findings are based on the best evidence. Others include poor studies and examine if design features influence results. There are arguments for

and against the various practices (Card, 2012). Regardless of how authors assess risk of bias and quality, they help establish reader confidence by explaining and justifying their decisions.

The next section in the protocol details data analysis and synthesis. Bates et al. mention they will consider conducting a meta-analysis if suitable data is obtained with subgroup analysis being guided by theory-based intervention characteristics. The PRISMA-P protocol requires a greater level of detail regarding quantitative analysis than PROSPERO. The difference may reflect that PRISMA-P is biased towards quantitative assessments of intervention effectiveness, whereas PROSPERO protocols are more flexible, allowing the inclusion of a greater variety of review methods and designs. To be more flexible, the questions need to be less specific in the information they demand.

Towards the end of the protocol, Bates et al. then record more administrative details, such as contact information, language, and country. Two useful features in these final sections include: (a) the dates of protocol registration and the publication of the latest version, and (b) amendment acknowledgment and justification. Both PROSPERO and PRISMA-P recognize that protocols sometimes need to be adjusted as researchers proceed with their projects.

Protocols are regarded as living documents that may be updated to reflect changes. Bates et al., for example, changed the time period within which included studies had to have been published, from 1995–2017 to 1990–2017, to avoid excluding a small number of relevant studies. As mentioned above, documenting changes helps to reduce reporting bias.

In addition to reporting dates of protocol registration and current version publication, PROSPERO also lists a summary of how much of the review has already been completed. These details indicate whether reviewers are still engaged in the project or if it has become dormant. Registering a review is relatively easy, free, and helps people stake their claim over a topic. Researchers who register, but do not complete reviews may be denying the community useful information, because other investigators, who would have completed the project, may decide against undertaking a synthesis. Bates et al. (in press), however, did complete and publish their project and the citation details are in the reference list if the topic is of interest.

Summary

One myth among sport, exercise, and physical activity academics and students is that systematic syntheses are just like any other review, just packaged to appear more scientific. These individuals may view systematic reviews as soft or easy publications. Their perceptions change once they embark on the process and realize the amount of work and attention to detail required. Ploughing through hundreds or thousands of hits from an electronic search, for example, can be soul-destroying, especially if you stumble across a previously unknown archive. Although nothing in life is guaranteed, it is helpful to ensure that if you start a project there is a better than even chance of finishing it. The purpose of this chapter has been to discuss factors to consider in planning a review so that the odds are in your favour.

❷ Learning Exercises

1. Visit the PROSPERO and Cochrane Collaboration online libraries and search for protocols on topics similar to your areas of interest. Compare and contrast the protocols, specifically asking yourself which of the two:
   - Is clearer and more coherent across the questions and methods.
   - Provides a greater level of detail in terms of data search, extraction, analysis, and synthesis.
   - Seems to have made better attempts to detail and justify amendments (if any).
   - Also, are there gaps in either of the protocols that lead you to doubt if the project will be completed.
   - For each protocol consider what changes you might have made and for what reasons.
2. Above, I have detailed the three stages involved in auditing systematic review competencies. Undertake the process for yourself. Start by identifying the necessary skills and knowledge, seeking advice from other sources if needed. Then complete ◘ Fig. 2.2. Based on your audit, identify ways that you can either

develop necessary competencies for yourself or people you can collaborate with who have these skills.

3. If you undertook exercise three in chapter one, then you have started to formulate a potential review question you could pursue as you read this book. Using the PRISMA-P structure presented in ◘ Table 2.1 begin developing a protocol, adding in as much detail as you can. Treat the protocol as a living document that you will develop and modify as you work your way through this book.

References

Arthur, A., & Hancock, B. (2009). *Introduction to the research process*. Nottingham and Shieffield: The NIHR RDS for the East Midlands/Yorkshire and the Humber.

Bates, G., Begley, E., Tod, D., Jones, L., Leavey, C., & McVeigh, J. (in press). A systematic review investigating the behaviour change strategies in interventions to prevent misuse of anabolic steroids. *Journal of Health Psychology*. ► https://doi.org/10.1177/1359105317737607.

Booth, A., Sutton, A., & Papaioannou, D. (2016). *Systematic approaches to a successful literature review* (2nd ed.). Thousand Oaks, CA: Sage.

Card, N. A. (2012). *Applied meta-analysis for social science research*. New York, NY: Guilford.

Ioannidis, J. P. A. (2016). The mass production of redundant, misleading, and conflicted systematic reviews and meta-analyses. *The Milbank Quarterly, 94*, 485–514. ► https://doi.org/10.1111/1468-0009.12210.

Jadad, A. R., Cook, D. J., & Browman, G. P. (1997). A guide to interpreting discordant systematic reviews. *Canadian Medical Association Journal, 156*, 1411–1416.

Long, L. (2014). Routine piloting in systematic reviews—A modified approach? *Systematic Reviews, 3*, article 77. ► https://doi.org/10.1186/2046-4053-3-77.

Mallett, R., Hagen-Zanker, J., Slater, R., & Duvendack, M. (2012). The benefits and challenges of using systematic reviews in international development research. *Journal of Development Effectiveness, 4*, 445–455. ► https://doi.org/10.1080/19439342.2012.711342.

Mesly, O. (2017). *Project feasibility: Tools for uncovering points of vulnerability*. London, UK: Taylor & Francis.

Moher, D., Shamseer, L., Clarke, M., Ghersi, D., Liberati, A., Petticrew, M., ... PRISMA-P Group. (2015). Preferred reporting items for systematic review and meta-analysis protocols (PRISMA-P) 2015 statement. *Systematic Reviews, 4*, article 1. ► https://doi.org/10.1186/2046-4053-4-1.

Page, M. J., McKenzie, J. E., & Forbes, A. (2013). Many scenarios exist for selective inclusion and reporting of results in randomized trials and systematic reviews. *Journal of Clinical Epidemiology, 66*, 524–537. ► https://doi.org/10.1016/j.jclinepi.2012.10.010.

Pawson, R., Greenhalgh, T., Harvey, G., & Walshe, K. (2004). *Realist synthesis: An introduction*. Manchester, UK: Economic and Social Research Council.

Pinker, S. (2015). *The sense of style: The thinking person's guide to writing in the 21st century*. London, UK: Penguin Books.

Pope, C., Mays, N., & Popay, J. (2007). *Synthesizing qualitative and quantitative health evidence: A guide to methods*. Maidenhead, UK: Open University Press.

Shamseer, L., Moher, D., Clarke, M., Ghersi, D., Liberati, A., Petticrew, M., ... PRISMA-P Group. (2015). Preferred reporting items for systematic review and meta-analysis protocols (PRISMA-P) 2015: Elaboration and explanation. *British Medical Journal, 349*, article 7647. ► https://doi.org/10.1136/bmj.g7647.

Stroup, D. F., Berlin, J. A., Morton, S. C., Olkin, I., Williamson, G. D., Rennie, D., ... Thacker, S. B. (2000). Meta-analysis of observational studies in epidemiology: A proposal for reporting. *Journal of the American Medical Association, 283*, 2008–2012. ► https://doi.org/10.1001/jama.283.15.2008.

Tong, A., Flemming, K., McInnes, E., Oliver, S., & Craig, J. (2012). Enhancing transparency in reporting the synthesis of qualitative research: ENTREQ. *BMC Medical Research Methodology, 12*, article 181. ► https://doi.org/10.1186/1471-2288-12-181.

Tricco, A. C., Cogo, E., Page, M. J., Polisena, J., Booth, A., Dwan, K., ... Moher, D. (2016). A third of systematic reviews changed or did not specify the primary outcome: A PROSPERO register study. *Journal of Clinical Epidemiology, 79*, 46–54. ► https://doi.org/10.1016/j.jclinepi.2016.03.025.

Defining Suitable Review Questions

© The Author(s) 2019
D. Tod, *Conducting Systematic Reviews in Sport, Exercise, and Physical Activity*,
https://doi.org/10.1007/978-3-030-12263-8_3

3

Learning Objectives

After reading this chapter, you should be able to:
- Detail the value of clear, well-structured, and specific review questions.
- Describe factors to consider when developing questions.
- Write clear, well-structured, informative, and specific review questions.
- Use tools and techniques for defining the scope of questions.

Introduction

When teaching about systematic reviews, I sometimes start by inflating a balloon and asking students to predict where it will go when I set it free. I do this multiple times and the balloon ends up in various places, although never far from where I am standing. Having established it is pointless to predict the balloon's final resting place, I then use Sellotape to attach the reinflated balloon to a straw, through which I thread a length of string. The string allows me to direct the balloon to wherever I want it to go. Students typically understand the metaphor's point: when you have a direction and a strategy, you make optimal use of your energy. This message applies to synthesizing research. Reviews cost time, money, and energy. To make most of these resources we need some string, or a clear purpose. In this chapter, I provide guidance on pointing your string in the right direction.

The Value of Clear Well-Structured Review Questions

Across our numerous disciplines in sport, exercise, and physical activity, researchers are interested in various types of questions, often focused on description, association, or causality. When investigators measure or describe a variable or phenomenon, such as football players' body fat percentages or a team's culture, they are asking descriptive questions. When researchers estimate the strength of relationships among variables, or predict one variable from another, they are asking association questions (e.g., calculating jump height from ground reaction forces). When exploring the influence of one variable on another, such as during a randomized controlled trial, scientists are examining causality. For example, examining the influence of a physical activity intervention on social behaviour in autistic individuals is a causality-based question. Just as these various types of questions drive primary research, they also guide systematic reviews. Some people believe that systematic reviews are limited to synthesizing randomized controlled trials (Petticrew, 2001). As discussed in ▶ Chapter 1, however, systematic reviews can be used for a variety of questions and evidence types. Understanding the typical questions that get asked in sport, exercise, and physical activity research can assist in developing suitable well-structured review purpose statements.

Richardson (2005, August 9) outlined the benefits of clear specific questions:
- They direct people towards the relevant information that will assist with their own and other's needs.
- They contribute to the identification of optimal data search, analysis, and synthesis strategies.

- They aid people in visualizing the forms that their answers might take. Understanding the likely content and structure of the answers helps to reverse engineer methods.
- They facilitate salubrious communication among colleagues and stakeholders.
- They allow research consumers to make sense of current knowledge and to compare and contrast multiple reviews.
- They help ensure knowledge advancement and reward investigator curiosity.

In addition to those benefits Richardson (2005, August 9) described, clarity and structure helps reviewers assess if their questions are feasible, meaningful, relevant, and worth answering (Pope, Mays, & Popay, 2007). Individuals can consider the following criteria to help them decide if the proposed question warrants attention:

- Can an answer be obtained with the available time and resources?
- In what ways will the likely findings make a meaningful contribution to knowledge?
- How will the review assist practitioners and decision makers in their daily lives?
- Will the benefits I gain outweigh those from other activities I will not be able to undertake?

Although the final question seems miserly, people typically have competing demands that they need to balance to fulfil their work responsibilities.

As an additional benefit, clarity and structure allow for coherence across the review questions, methods, answers, and interpretations. A common example of incoherence involves confusing correlation with causality. Reviewers sometimes unintentionally slip into the language of causality when discussing descriptive research. As another example of incoherency, qualitative researchers sometimes think quantitatively, such as arguing that two variables are related when their data are focused on participants' perceptions about how two concepts vary. Correlations and people's perceptions about how concepts vary are each worthy of being examined, and doing so can advance knowledge and assist decision-making. These questions, however, are not the same as each other. Researchers sometimes overinterpret their findings (such as implying causality or correlation) because they want to emphasize the value of their work. But investigators do not have to imply that their results are more than they are, if they have asked relevant, meaningful questions. Instead, overinterpretation or speculation may distract readers from the study's contribution. Coherence can be enhanced by posing clear, well-defined, and specific questions, because they provide criteria against which reviewers can evaluate in their projects.

Factors Influencing the Development of Review Questions

Theoretical framework   Theoretical frameworks describe people's understanding of their interest areas and underpinning assumptions (Oliver, Dickerson, Bangpan, & Newman, 2017). Theoretical frameworks guide thinking regarding what questions are worth asking and how they can be answered. Systematic reviews have sometimes been criticized for being atheoretical (Petticrew, 2001). More accurately, however,

3

investigators do not always disclose, or are sometimes unaware of, their guiding frameworks. Researchers aware of their guiding frameworks can construct high quality coherent reviews by design rather than chance.

To illustrate, in their meta-analysis on deliberate practice and sporting expertise, Macnamara, Moreau, and Hambrick (2016) outlined the content-specific dimension to their theoretical framework: that expertise varies across individuals and is influenced by many factors. Within this framework, they estimated the strength of the association between deliberate practice and performance, and they assessed the influence of participant, task, and methodological moderators. Similar to many quantitative reviewers, however, they largely did not detail their epistemological, ontological, axiological, methodological, and confusingological assumptions, although they operated from a positivistic/post-positivistic framework (Yilmaz, 2013). Reviewers operating from qualitative perspectives often detail explicitly their philosophical assumptions, because their work's credibility is likely to be contested in the publication submission process.

Review purpose   Reviewers conduct their projects to advance knowledge, to assist real world decision-making, or both, and these purposes influence driving questions. When focused on knowledge advancement, investigators may have the freedom to pose focused and theoretically driven questions. Reviewers may have the freedom in this case to narrow their attention to specialized topics. In contrast, if the review is designed to support policy or decision-making, investigators may find their narrow questions are less suitable. Policymakers, for example, typically need answers to less straightforward questions. Their needs might be best informed by a series of interrelated questions. The difference between intervention efficacy and effectiveness provides an illustration. An efficacy or knowledge-based question might be "what is the influence of creatine supplementation on muscle mass retention in elderly individuals?" An effectiveness or decision support-based question could be "does this specific supplementation regime lead to muscle retention in the real world, given the uncontrollable factors that influence adherence?" Investigators who define clearly the purpose of their reviews are better able to encapsulate the objectives in clear questions.

Resource availability   When undertaking complex projects like systematic reviews, people often experience delusional optimism (Lovallo & Kahneman, 2003): the overestimation of benefits and underestimation of costs. Delusional optimism implies that the time, energy, resources, and costs needed to complete systematic syntheses will probably be greater than estimated, especially if undertaken by novice reviewers. To help increase planning accuracy, it is useful to adopt an outsider's perspective (Lovallo & Kahneman, 2003). Rather than focussing solely on their own expertise, time, and resource availability, researchers compare their proposed reviews with a range of similar projects. Benchmarking your project against others improves accuracy in determining a review's multiple costs, and assists in identifying answerable or feasible questions. With experience, teams will be able to benchmark their proposed projects against those they have recently completed.

Stakeholders Throughout the twentieth century there has been a move towards greater stakeholder involvement in science, leading to participatory research designs (Lincoln, Lynham, & Guba, 2018), where the power over a study's purpose, design, implementation, and dissemination is distributed among investigators and the communities with whom they work. This movement applies to systematic reviews, as much as primary research, because synthesis findings inform public policy (Rees & Oliver, 2017). Interacting with stakeholders maximizes the possibility that guiding questions are tailored towards decision support and that findings will have an influence in society. Involving stakeholders can add challenges and tensions to the review process (Boote, Baird, & Sutton, 2011). In recognition of the possible challenges, researchers have generated guidelines for involving the public in the review process, such as providing adequate training and engaging in regular reflection (Bayliss et al., 2016).

Phenomenon complexity Reviewers' areas of interest are often complex and even seemingly simple questions may disguise multifaceted phenomena. The UK Medical Research Council, for example, has discussed ways interventions vary, such as the (a) number of and interactions among components within the different groups, (b) number and difficulty of intervention personnel and recipient behaviours, (c) number of targeted population groups and levels, (d) number and variability of outcomes, and (e) degree of intervention flexibility (Craig et al., 2008). In a similar fashion, the ways that non-intervention or descriptive studies differ include discrepancies in operational definitions, measurement techniques, underpinning philosophy, number of and categorization of variables (e.g., predictor, criterion, moderator, and mediator), participants, and contexts.

Heterogeneity is a key issue, as illustrated in the lumping versus splitting debate (Squires, Valentine, & Grimshaw, 2013). *Splitters* suggest only highly similar studies can combined, whereas *lumpers* argue minor differences are not important and investigations should be pooled unless there are strong countering reasons. Squires et al. advocated lumping studies where possible, because it reduces bias, decreases the occurrence of chance findings, and allows results to be assessed across a range of contexts, populations, and variables. Following up a general examination with subgroup scrutiny or sensitivity analysis, as often done in meta-analyses, represents a compromise. Guidance exists on when to combine and separate studies (Squires et al., 2013), but more generally, investigators can ask themselves:

- How much lumping or splitting is needed to answer the question?
- To what degree can they rationalize splitting or lumping the evidence?
- What assistance does underlying theory provide?

Scoping the evidence and developing theoretical frameworks can help answer these questions.

Extent of the literature Although it sounds like a bad joke, a common question is "how many studies are needed to do a systematic review?" The punchline is "zero," because systematic reviewing is a process, not an output. A rigorous search that returns no studies is still a systematic review and demonstrates that there is no evidence on which to answer the question (Petticrew & Roberts, 2006). The question, however, is not meaningful. The substantive question is "how many studies are needed to produce a review that the intended audience will accept?" The answer is, "it depends." In some situations, it may be necessary to know that no research has been undertaken, such as when making decisions about intervening in people's lives. In other situations, a review that includes multiple studies may be considered inadequate. For example, journal editors may reject reviews on the basis of too few studies, if they believe the resultant knowledge will be of insufficient interest to the readership. At the other end of the scale, sometimes there is too much literature to synthesize meaningfully, a state of affairs that probably occurs most often if reviewers fail to narrow their questions sufficiently or adequately define their topics of interest. In a configural review, for example, if investigators have not defined the scope of relevant research, they may be able to justify the inclusion of evermore studies because they help broaden or deepen the developing theory until it resembles a unified theory of everything. These theories, however, are at risk of being too vague in their predictions to be helpful.

Nevertheless, some guidance can be offered (Petticrew & Roberts, 2006). First, ask informed individuals, such as content and methodological experts, what they think might be acceptable. Second, avoid overselling the findings, but be honest about the review's scope and limitations. Ensure conclusions are commensurate with the evidence. Third, highlight the review's contribution to knowledge and decision support. Fourth, when developing the project, undertake a scoping review to gain insight into the evidence-base and adjust the review's scope, questions, and methods to find a balance that audiences will accept (most often this will involve narrowing down the question).

Components of Clear Review Purpose Statements

Authors help themselves and readers by making their purpose statements clear and explicit. To enhance clarity, it is also helpful to set the purpose apart from other sections in the introduction by giving it a new paragraph. The paragraph may also include any working definitions of relevant terms to assist readers in understanding the purpose, and factors that delimit the review's scope. Specific research questions and hypotheses may also be presented if relevant. Creswell (2014) provided useful advice on developing quantitative, qualitative, and mixed-method primary research questions. His advice is relevant for systematic reviews.

Quantitative purpose statements   Quantitative research involves the numerical measurement of operationally defined variables that represent constructs. These numbers allow researchers to (a) describe participants or objects according to those variables, (b) examine how groups of people or things differ from each other, and (c) explore how variables relate, predict, and interact with each other. Quantitative questions are infused with these ideas of measurement, relationships, and causality. Components of clear quantitative questions include (Creswell, 2014):

- Words such as "purpose," "objective," and "aim" that indicate authors' review goals.
- Declaring the type of systematic review being undertaken (e.g., meta-analysis, economic evaluation).
- The variables to be examined, along with an indication of what type they may be, such as independent, dependent, predictor, criterion, mediator, or moderator.
- A description of how the variables relate to each other.
- Positioning variables in a logical fashion, such as putting predictor or independent before criterion or dependent variables.
- Acknowledging the design of included studies if they are similar.
- Stating the participant groups and research settings included.

The discussion around the purpose statement may also include the theoretical framework underpinning the review and operational definitions of the variables. In practice, it is unlikely that published review purpose statements will contain all of these features, but clear explicit ones will have most of them. To illustrate, a review purpose might read:

» The purpose (*signalling the purpose statement*) of this meta-analysis (*review type*) is to draw on randomized controlled trials (*type of included studies*) to estimate the influence (*how the variables relate to each other*) that weight training frequency (*independent variable*), compared with no training, has on maximal strength performance (*dependent variable*) in elderly people who have not previously trained with weights (*participant group*). For the current review, elderly people were defined as individuals over the age of 65 (*defining relevant terms*) ...

Qualitative purpose statements   Qualitative research differs from its quantitative counterpart in its language, focus, and philosophical underpinnings. Given these differences, review purpose statements need to be structured differently. Whereas quantitative research seeks to measure variables and their relationships with each other, qualitative investigations aim to describe how people perceive and portray their social and physical worlds. Clear explicit review statements include (Creswell, 2014):

- Words such as "purpose," "objective," and "aim" that indicate authors' review goals.
- Declaring the type of systematic review being undertaken (e.g., meta-ethnography, realist synthesis).
- The phenomenon of interest.
- An action verb that describes what the reviewer is hoping to achieve, such as "explore," "describe," or "identify".
- Non-directional language to avoid bias towards particular outcomes.
- Acknowledging the research design of included studies if similar.
- Stating the participant groups and research settings included.

As mentioned with quantitative questions, the paragraph in which the purpose statement resides may also include the theoretical framework underpinning the review and detail working definitions of relevant terms. Similarly, although published qualitative review purpose statements may not have all the above features, it is likely they will have several of them. To illustrate, a qualitative review statement might read:

» The purpose (*signalling the purpose statement*) of this meta-study (*review type*) is to draw on qualitative investigations (*type of included studies*) to explore (*action verb*) how primary school children (*participant group*) understand the benefits of compulsory physical education (*phenomenon of interest*). To assist readers not familiar with the UK education system, primary school children are aged (*defining relevant terms*) …

Mixed-study reviews   Mixed-study reviews combine qualitative, quantitative, and mixed-method research. Example ways these studies can be synthesized include the convergent, sequential explanatory, sequential exploratory, or parallel designs (see ▶ Chapter 9 on data analysis, Pluye & Hong, 2014). Guidelines on developing purpose statements include (Creswell, 2014):

— Signal the purpose statement with phrases such as "the purpose of this review …"
— Indicate the content area of the review to help readers understand the topic of interest.
— Declare the type of mixed-study design.
— Explain the reason for including both qualitative and quantitative evidence.
— If using a sequential design, follow-up with specific questions for each phase.

As above, the paragraph in which the purpose statement resides may include the theoretical framework and working definitions. Published mixed-study review purpose statements may not have all the above features, but good ones will have several. To illustrate:

» The purpose (*signalling purpose statement*) of this sequential exploratory mixed-study review (*review type*) was to examine the types and correlates of same gender sexual harassment that female athletes experience (*content area*). In phase 1, we used thematic content analysis on existing qualitative research to generate the various types of same gender sexual harassment female athletes have reported. In phase two, our framework was used to generate frequencies and correlates of the types of same gender sexual harassment reported in quantitative surveys (*follow-up questions*). By undertaking a mixed-study review, we were able to ensure that the types of incidents were not limited to those predetermined by quantitative surveyors, but were informed by athletes' own reports (*explaining the need for a mixed-study approach*). We defined same gender sexual harassment as … (*defining jargon*).

Useful Tools

Question mnemonics   You may have realized that systematic reviewers adore checklists, proformas, and mnemonics. There are sounds reasons for their use: human memory is fallible. Mnemonics help reviewers identify the features of clear specific questions. These mnemonics can ensure coherency across a review. In addition to assisting with question clarity and structure, these mnemonics can also guide method construction, such as helping to identify search terms, items for data extraction, and suitable analysis procedures.

PICO is one such mnemonic frequently discussed in systematic review literature and stands for *Population, Intervention, Comparison,* and *Outcome.* It is suited for reviews of intervention research. For example, PICO might lead to the following:

- *Population*: The purpose of the review is to assess in asymptomatic male adolescents …
- *Intervention*: the influence of high-intensity interval training …
- *Comparison*: compared with continuous endurance training …
- *Outcomes*: on blood pressure, body fat levels, and heart rate.

There are various adaptions such as PICOT and PICOTT, where the Ts stand for *Time, Type of question,* and *Type of study* (Davies, 2011).

Researchers have proposed numerous mnemonics. For example, SPIDER is suggested for qualitative research (Cooke, Smith, & Booth, 2012), and stands for *Sample, Phenomenon of Interest, Design, Evaluation,* and *Research.* For example:

- *Sample*: How do team sport athletes …
- *Phenomenon of Interest*: describe sporting culture …
- *Design*: during informal interviews and interactions with other players …
- *Evaluation*: as perceived by researchers acting as participant observers …
- *Research*: during ethnographic studies.

There are mnemonics for various subject areas and study designs. The mnemonic FINER is a generic example for establishing good research questions and highlights the criteria of *Feasible, Interesting, Novel, Ethical,* and *Relevant* (Hulley, Cummings, Browner, Grady, & Newman, 2013). These frameworks, however, are tools to help reviewers define and structure their questions. They are not laws that need to be followed slavishly. It would be acceptable to tailor a mnemonic to suit an individual's needs.

Visual representations   Visual representations may assist in developing theoretical frameworks within which to identify, locate, and prioritize review questions. Examples include mind maps, concept maps, flowcharts, logic models, and diagrams. These graphical methods can be particularly helpful when the phenomenon of interest is complex, by detailing the key components and their relationships (Booth, Sutton, & Papaioannou, 2016).

To illustrate, Williams and Andersen (1998) presented in pictorial form their stress response and athletic injury theory to suggest how psychosocial variables influenced sports injury occurrence. The model was the basis for a meta-analytic review (Ivarsson et al., 2017), helping the authors identify and prioritize two questions. First, what are the psychosocial predictors of sports injury? Second, what was the influence of psychological interventions on injury rates? Visual representations can be expanded or shrunk to suit the authors' preferences, such as making them large enough to be able to include the evidence or list the research underpinning each aspect of the model. Similar to the question mnemonics discussed above, visual presentations are tools that can be modified to help reviewers formalize their thinking.

Chapter Case Example: Creatine Supplementation and Upper Limb Strength Performance

Lanhers et al. (2017) examined creatine supplementation's influence on upper limb strength. Their review illustrates material discussed in the current chapter. The paper appeared in *Sports Medicine*, volume 47, pages 163–173. Their purpose statement (p. 164) contains several of Creswell's (2014) features presented above:

We aimed to conduct (*phrase signalling intention*) a systematic review and meta-analyses (*type of review*) of RCTs (*detailing type of included studies*) comparing the effects (*suggesting how the variables might relate*) of creatine supplementation (*independent variable*) and placebo (*control condition*) on upper limb strength performance (*dependent variable*) measured after exercises of less than 3 min in duration. The meta-analyses were stratified by muscles or groups of muscles.

Notice also the logical ordering of the variables, starting with the independent and leading to the dependent; and additional information about the stratification of analyses. The purpose statement provides readers with clear insight into the review's direction. If the question was to conform to the PICO mnemonic, the authors might have detailed the type of participants used in the studies, although this is mentioned in first paragraph of the method ("healthy males or females, independent of age …").

The purpose statement sits well within Lanhers et al.'s (2017) theoretical framework discussed in the introduction. Regarding the framework's content, the authors discuss the physiological theory explaining why creatine is expected to influence strength performance. Lanhers et al. also reveal their assumptions underpinning the research process, and it is clear they reside within a positivist/post-positivist orientation, as detailed by their reference to randomized controlled trials being the "highest level of proof," the need for placebo controls, and use of causal language. There is a coherent match between the theoretical framework and question, illustrating the type of approach that would be typically used in physiological research examining the effects of a dietary supplement on biological variables.

The coherency continues through the methods section. For example, the inclusion criteria featured details consistent with the purpose statement (e.g., description of the strength measure), theoretical orientation (e.g., reference to double blinded RCTs), and type of review (e.g., reference to statistical information). Taken together, the article's opening stanzas present a theoretical orientation, well-structured question, and level of coherency that engages interested readers and leaves them wanting to learn more, a feat not achieved in all systematic reviews.

Summary

It is understandable that the compass is a common analogy when discussing review questions. Just as compasses point hikers along their desired journeys, review questions orient investigators and readers to the project's direction. If you search for a compass on Amazon, you will face a deluge of options and learn that their customer ratings vary considerably, implying that some do a better job than others. Similarly, there are endless ways to present review questions, but some are more useful than others. In the current chapter, I have discussed the various benefits of having clear well-worded purpose statements and provided advice on their construction. If you decide to buy a compass from a bricks and mortar store, your selection might be influenced by the packaging. Marketers know that pretty boxes make a difference. There are two dimensions to the packaging of review questions. First, questions surrounded by an explicit coherent theoretical framework are often easier to understand than when not packaged well. Second, review questions are typically placed at the end of the introduction and benefit from being in a well-to-do neighbourhood. In the next chapter, I will discuss how to use introductions to set the scene and justify the purpose statement and the review in general.

❓ Learning Exercises

1. Find a quantitative systematic review in an area of interest, read it, and then answer the following questions:
   - How well does the purpose address Creswell's (2014) features discussed above?
   - Can you identify the guiding theoretical framework?
   - What is your assessment regarding the coherency of the paper across its purpose, method, analysis, and interpretation?
2. Repeat the first learning exercise using a review that synthesized qualitative research.
3. If you undertook the exercises in chapters one and two, then you are well on the way to creating your review. Taking your protocol, revisit the question in light of the current chapter. Make changes to ensure that the purpose statement conforms to the guidance detailed above. Begin to consider how the changes you have made might influence the method.

References

Bayliss, K., Starling, B., Raza, K., Johansson, E. C., Zabalan, C., Moore, S., ... Stack, R. (2016). Patient involvement in a qualitative meta-synthesis: Lessons learnt. *Research Involvement and Engagement, 2*, article 18. ▶ https://doi.org/10.1186/s40900-016-0032-0.

Boote, J., Baird, W., & Sutton, A. (2011). Public involvement in the systematic review process in health and social care: A narrative review of case examples. *Health Policy, 102*, 105–116. ▶ https://doi.org/10.1016/j.healthpol.2011.05.002.

Booth, A., Sutton, A., & Papaioannou, D. (2016). *Systematic approaches to a successful literature review* (2nd ed.). Thousand Oaks, CA: Sage.

Cooke, A., Smith, D., & Booth, A. (2012). Beyond PICO: The SPIDER tool for qualitative evidence synthesis. *Qualitative Health Research, 22*, 1435–1443. ▶ https://doi.org/10.1177/1049732312452938.

Craig, P., Dieppe, P., Macintyre, S., Michie, S., Nazareth, I., & Petticrew, M. (2008). Developing and evaluating complex interventions: The new Medical Research Council guidance. *British Medical Journal, 337*, article 1655. ▶ https://doi.org/10.1136/bmj.a1655.

Creswell, J. W. (2014). *Research design: Qualitative, quantitative, and mixed methods approaches* (4th ed.). Thousand Oaks, CA: Sage.

Davies, K. S. (2011). Formulating the evidence based practice question: A review of the frameworks. *Evidence Based Library and Information Practice, 6*, 75–80.

Hulley, S. B., Cummings, S. R., Browner, W. S., Grady, D. G., & Newman, T. B. (2013). *Designing clinical research* (4th ed.). Philadelphia, PA: Lippincott Williams & Wilkins.

Ivarsson, A., Johnson, U., Andersen, M. B., Tranaeus, U., Stenling, A., & Lindwall, M. (2017). Psychosocial factors and sport injuries: Meta-analyses for prediction and prevention. *Sports Medicine, 47*, 353–365. ► https://doi.org/10.1007/s40279-016-0578-x.

Lanhers, C., Pereira, B., Naughton, G., Trousselard, M., Lesage, F. X., & Dutheil, F. (2017). Creatine supplementation and upper limb strength performance: A systematic review and meta-analysis. *Sports Medicine, 47*, 163–173. ► https://doi.org/10.1007/s40279-016-0571-4.

Lincoln, Y. S., Lynham, S. A., & Guba, E. G. (2018). Paradigmatic controversies, contradictions, and emerging confluences, revisited. In N. K. Denzin & Y. S. Lincoln (Eds.), *The Sage handbook of qualitative research* (5th ed., pp. 108–150). Thousand Oaks, CA: Sage.

Lovallo, D., & Kahneman, D. (2003). Delusions of success. *Harvard Business Review, 81*, 56–63.

Macnamara, B. N., Moreau, D., & Hambrick, D. Z. (2016). The relationship between deliberate practice and performance in sports: A meta-analysis. *Perspectives on Psychological Science, 11*, 333–350. ► https://doi.org/10.1177/1745691616635591.

Oliver, S., Dickerson, K., Bangpan, M., & Newman, M. (2017). Getting started with a review. In D. Gough, S. Oliver, & J. Thomas (Eds.), *An introduction to systematic reviews* (2nd ed., pp. 71–92). Thousand Oaks, CA: Sage.

Petticrew, M. (2001). Systematic reviews from astronomy to zoology: Myths and misconceptions. *British Medical Journal, 322*, 98–101. ► https://doi.org/10.1136/bmj.322.7278.98.

Petticrew, M., & Roberts, H. (2006). *Systematic reviews in the social sciences: A practical guide*. Malden, MA: Blackwell.

Pluye, P., & Hong, Q. N. (2014). Combining the power of stories and the power of numbers: Mixed methods research and mixed studies reviews. *Annual Review of Public Health, 35*, 29–45. ► https://doi.org/10.1146/annurev-publhealth-032013-182440.

Pope, C., Mays, N., & Popay, J. (2007). *Synthesizing qualitative and quantitative health evidence: A guide to methods*. Maidenhead, UK: Open University Press.

Rees, R., & Oliver, S. (2017). Stakeholder perspectives and participation in reviews. In D. Gough, S. Oliver, & J. Thomas (Eds.), *An introduction to systematic reviews* (2nd ed., pp. 19–41). Thousand Oaks, CA: Sage.

Richardson, S. (2005, August 9). Focus on questions [Web log comment]. Retrieved from ► https://www.jiscmail.ac.uk/cgi-bin/webadmin?A2=ind0508&L=EVIDENCE-BASED-HEALTH&F=&S=&P=10841.

Squires, J. E., Valentine, J. C., & Grimshaw, J. M. (2013). Systematic reviews of complex interventions: Framing the review question. *Journal of Clinical Epidemiology, 66*, 1215–1222. ► https://doi.org/10.1016/j.jclinepi.2013.05.013.

Williams, J. M., & Andersen, M. B. (1998). Psychosocial antecedents of sport injury: Review and critique of the stress and injury model. *Journal of Applied Sport Psychology, 10*, 5–25. ► https://doi.org/10.1080/10413209808406375.

Yilmaz, K. (2013). Comparison of quantitative and qualitative research traditions: Epistemological, theoretical, and methodological differences. *European Journal of Education, 48*, 311–325. ► https://doi.org/10.1111/ejed.12014.

Justifying the Review

D. Tod, *Conducting Systematic Reviews in Sport, Exercise, and Physical Activity*,
https://doi.org/10.1007/978-3-030-12263-8_4

Learning Objectives

After reading this chapter, you should be able to:
- Detail the objectives of systematic review introductions.
- Develop a well-structured review introduction.
- Differentiate configurative and aggregative review introductions.

Introduction

4

In the previous chapter, I mentioned the value of a compass when hiking and drew parallels with the purpose statement in a systematic review. When hiking, a map complements a compass, and together these two tools help individuals reach their destinations. Maps provide hikers with a representation of the landscapes they will pass through. The introduction in a systematic review also provides a tailored representation of the knowledge landscape in which the project is located. The accuracy of a map is influenced by cartographer's expertise and knowledge of the terrain. Similarly, the introduction in a systematic synthesis is influenced by reviewers' understanding of the content area, and their expertise will have a bearing on how well the section helps readers understand existing knowledge, the direction the project will take, and the value of the resulting information. In the current chapter, I discuss how the introduction forms a stylized map that helps justify the review. I then provide guidance on how to construct an introduction that sets up the rest of the review.

The Introduction's Objectives

Introductions have three primary aims (Kendall, Silk, & Chu, 2000). First, engage the audience and interest them sufficiently that they read the document. Second, draw on background information to provide a rationale for doing the review. Third, demonstrate how the review will contribute to knowledge and provide information to support decision-making. These three challenging tasks are made more or less difficult depending on the context in which the work occurs. Introductions in reviews slated for academic journal publication, for example, may have freedom to emphasise the knowledge advancement benefits and may give limited attention to practical implications. Introductions in reviews sponsored by external funders may lack an emphasis on knowledge advancement, but instead highlight the ways the project will meet the stakeholder's needs and assist in policy or decision-making. In the second case, the introduction may include few references, if any, to current knowledge. Systematic reviews may also appear in master's or doctoral dissertations. Typically, space is not a limitation and students have opportunities to expand on arguments fully to justify their work. In addition to justifying their work, students also need to demonstrate to a marker that they understand the type of project they are undertaking and that they have a broader understanding of the topic. As a result, dissertation introductions might cover more literature than would be included in a journal publication. Also, students may provide more details about the systematic review process to show they have command of the method's relevance for their subject.

For researchers and postgraduate students, emphasizing the ways that their reviews further knowledge is a key criterion by which their work is evaluated. In convincing others that their projects are worthy, these individuals may come across the perception that reviewing is derivative work or is second rate research (Chalmers, Hedges, & Cooper, 2002). Such perceptions are changing, because there is greater acknowledgement of the limitations with individual studies. There is also a realization that combining the results of various studies can lead to new knowledge or greater theoretical understanding. Meta-analyses, for example, provide estimates of effect sizes with greater precision than those presented in individual studies. Qualitative approaches to systematic reviewing can provide greater breadth and depth to theory than achieved by single qualitative investigations.

The increasing value of systematic reviews is illustrated in the hierarchy of evidence that ranks research designs by their internal validity (Chalmers et al., 2002). Systematic reviews reside at the apex of the hierarchy. The hierarchy of evidence is not applicable for all knowledge areas, however, such as those topics where intervention research is infeasible, unethical, or unable to answer the questions being asked. Nevertheless, it does help people appreciate that reviewing is a valuable task. Although reviews are receiving greater appreciation, it is still incumbent on investigators to explicitly detail the ways in which their work advances knowledge or helps people live their lives.

There are several ways that reviews can contribute to knowledge (Booth, Sutton, & Papaioannou, 2016). First, a review can challenge existing beliefs and understandings, especially where people have been guided by limited access to evidence or have held personal assumptions about an area. Smith and Glass' (1977) meta-analysis, for example, challenged the beliefs about the ineffectiveness of psychotherapy that were common in the 1970s by revealing that such interventions were helpful for clients. Second, systematic reviews can resolve academic disputes and disagreements. For example, people have disagreed over the effects that competitive environments have on performance across domains, including sport. In their review, Murayama and Elliot (2012) revealed that competition has indirect effects on performance that are mediated by whether it encourages approach or avoidance goals. Third, reviews can introduce new, or revitalize dormant, lines of research by providing new or improved perspectives on phenomena. One advantage of meta-analyses, for example, is that they provide the best, and most up-to-date, estimate of an effect size and its precision, such as the influence of an intervention on an outcome or the strength and direction of a relationship between two variables (Borenstein, Hedges, Higgins, & Rothstein, 2009).

Configurative Versus Aggregative Reviews

In ▶ Chapter 1, I introduced configurative and aggregative reviews. I will discuss the differences between the two in more detail in ▶ Chapter 9, because of the implications for data analysis. Nevertheless, some understanding of these two types of review helps with writing the introduction. Although I have presented them as different, configuration and aggregation are not mutually exclusive, but reside at opposite ends of a continuum. Reviews often have elements of both to a greater or lesser extent (Gough & Thomas, 2017).

Configurative reviews assemble the evidence, piecing it together to form an answer to the review question (Gough & Thomas, 2017). These reviews often focus on theory development. They strive to explore and interpret data in new ways, typically using heterogeneous primary research. Think of individuals using Lego blocks of different shapes, sizes, and colours to build new creations. Configurative reviews may include interpretative and inductive elements.

Aggregative reviews involve piling up, stacking, or adding together findings from research to test theory, hypotheses, or answer questions (Gough & Thomas, 2017). Data is normally collated from homogenous studies to gain greater precision and confidence in the findings. Univariate meta-analyses exemplify aggregative reviews.

The configurative-aggregative continuum is not a proxy for the qualitative and quantitative divide (Thomas, O'Mara-Eves, Harden, & Newman, 2017). Although aggregative reviews often pile up quantitative findings, they may also stack together qualitative results in a manner similar to a thematic content analysis. Similarly, configurative reviews may piece together new knowledge or develop theory based on quantitative results, as is done when researchers employ multivariate or structural equation modelling meta-analytic techniques. Nevertheless, awareness of the configuration-aggregation continuum can help authors provide a rationale for their reviews. To illustrate, people undertaking configural reviews can pitch their justifications along the lines of theory generation or development. They might argue they are seeking to provide novel ways of understanding the phenomenon of interest. They are searching for enlightenment. In contrast, individuals undertaking aggregative reviews may argue they are testing theory to help assess its robustness and the level of confidence we can have in the knowledge. Aggregative reviews also contribute to knowledge specificity and precision.

Possible Introduction Structure

Although there is no set formula for structuring introductions, they often start by positioning the research area within a broad context, and then summarize existing knowledge, before narrowing the focus on the current study (Kendall et al., 2000). Students are sometimes taught that the introduction is where they should "review the literature," but this advice is woolly. The introduction is not a review of literature, and even less so in a systematic synthesis. Introductions are where authors explain the purpose of, and justify, their projects. Introductions are dissimilar to UK ordnance survey maps that are highly detailed and present everything in the landscape. Instead, review introductions, especially those for external funders and journal publication, typically detail just enough of existing knowledge to explain why the project is worth undertaking. Although they do discuss existing knowledge, reference to literature serves the purpose of rationalizing the study.

One helpful template for structuring an introduction is the deficiencies model illustrated in ◻ Fig. 4.1 (Creswell, 2014). The approach starts broad and narrows down to the specific purpose statements through a series of five steps, presented as separate questions in ◻ Fig. 4.1. By answering the five questions, writers are including relevant

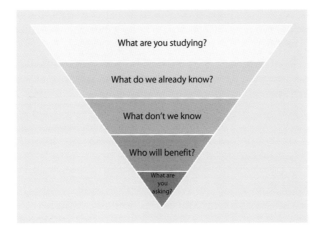

□ Fig. 4.1 Creswell's (2014) deficiencies model for an introduction

content in a logical structure that helps readers position the review questions within the broader topic area and appreciate why they deserve to be addressed. Creswell's model is a generic and recognizable template. Once familiar with the structure, you will recognize it in many systematic reviews and primary research publications.

First, what are you studying? The opening gambit is where authors catch readers' attention and set the research area within a broad, often social, context. There are various hooks by which readers can be reeled in, including striking statistics, demonstrating relevance to everyday life, asking rhetorical questions, using analogies, drawing on historical facts, or emphasizing a lack of research (Kendall et al., 2000). Strategies can be combined to fashion highly attractive lures. In developing the opening sentences, Bem (2004) suggested avoiding jargon, easing readers into the topic area, using examples to illustrate abstract material, and focusing on people rather than research. To illustrate these suggestions, read the following two opening sentences to a review article and decide which attracts your interest more than the other:

» *First example:* Since their appearance, Pope et al.'s seminal articles, along with their book, *The Adonis Complex*, have sparked research on muscle dysmorphia. Their work did not occur in a vacuum, however, and other researchers around a similar and earlier time were investigating the role a perceived lack of muscularity could play in individuals' (mostly males) lives.

» *Second example*: Males differ radically in their anxiety levels about their body shapes, with many being sufficiently anxious about their lack of muscle that they risk their health and wellbeing through drug abuse, excessive exercise, and risky diets. These unhappy individuals also experience broken relationships and employment difficulties. Empathetic sport psychologists ask: how do we help these men?

Most individuals suggest example two attracts their interest more than the first one. The first example is from a published article (Tod, Edwards, & Cranswick, 2016), but suffers because the focus is on what researchers have done, rather than the people whose lives have been examined. (Most readers are not interested in how researchers spend their time.) The second example, however, avoids jargon, focuses on people, and highlights the detrimental influence on men's health and well-being. Notice also the rhetorical question which encourages readers to become active and provide an answer. Having caught readers in their net, authors can move to the second element.

4

Second, what do we already know?   The American Psychological Association (2010, p. 28) suggests authors should "discuss the relevant related literature, but do not feel compelled to include an exhaustive historical account." There is a balance to be struck: to justify a systematic synthesis writers need to overview current knowledge, but in a way that avoids producing a literature review. One strategy is to identify the golden thread that runs throughout the entire systematic review and begin weaving it in the introduction. Authors can start by encapsulating the golden thread in the purpose statement and then ask themselves how they can flesh out the idea to clarify why the review was justified in being undertaken.

Another strategy is to consider the rationale for the review, and then base the introduction around this justification. For example, if the justification is to resolve a conflict, authors can structure existing knowledge around the various sides to the debate. As another example, if reviewers hope to introduce or revitalize an avenue of inquiry, they might present existing knowledge in a way that reveals the gaping hole in understanding. Basing the literature around the review's justification provides a tidy transition into the third section of the introduction, as discussed below.

Abstract stacking is one writing strategy to avoid, and involves focusing on studies one at a time, often presenting details that do not help reviewers justify their projects (Kendall et al., 2000). Extreme examples of abstract stacking read like a series of high school book reports with no clear link between paragraphs or any apparent overall direction. Sometimes there is a need to discuss an individual piece of work, but these articles are normally central to the review's topic and even then only the essential features are mentioned. A stronger writing strategy is to integrate studies and highlight their commonalities or differences, either in terms of content or method.

Although "citation of and specific credit to relevant earlier works are signs of scientific and scholarly responsibility and are essential for the growth of a cumulative science" (APA, 2010, p. 28), there are limited benefits to padding the introduction or reference list with irrelevant citations. Concise well-structured introductions, based around just the key references, demonstrate greater understanding and critical thought than lengthy meandering ones bloated with citations.

Third, what do we not know?   This question is a flippant way of asking about the deficiencies in current knowledge. In primary research, it is common to argue that the proposed study is justified because it has not been conducted previously. The argument, however, provides insufficient grounds to rationalize an investigation (or a review). For example, a study might not have been undertaken previously because it is not worth doing. The argument is incomplete and researchers who outline the knowledge and real-world benefits from doing the study provide a stronger rationale. For example, arguing that a study is using white rats, because they have not yet been examined and all previous research has used brown rats is not a compelling justification. Instead, the author might explain the ways in which white and brown rats differ, and how these variations make it uncertain that theory about one group transfers to the other. The author can then argue that a study on white rats makes it possible to evaluate the generalizability or robustness of current theory.

Review authors sometimes invoke a similar rationale by arguing that a particular area of research has not yet been reviewed. They may even justify a systematic review in a similar way. A review, however, is not justifiable because it is a systematic synthesis, even if the first of its kind. A systematic review is justified by way it contributes, such as extending knowledge, challenging theory, or informing policy and practice. Authors provide stronger rationales by showing how their work helps to remodel the landscape rather than just filling in a hole. Yes, filling holes does remodel the landscape, but it is up to authors to show how.

There are various ways reviewers can explain the deficiencies in current knowledge. First, they might identify methodological flaws in previous reviews that cast doubt on the findings and then show how their work will address these limitations. Second, authors can discuss the limited scope of previous syntheses and explain how they are going to extent boundaries. To illustrate, if new primary research has appeared since a previous review, then an updated synthesis may add to knowledge. Third, reviewers might argue that the use of a previously untested theoretical perspective may generate new insights to a phenomenon. Realist syntheses (see ▶ Chapter 1), for example, compliment reviews that establish whether or not an intervention works, because they flesh out "what works for whom, in what circumstances, in what respects, and how" (Pawson, Greenhalgh, Harvey, & Walshe, 2004, p. V)?

Fourth, who will benefit?   If authors have identified the deficiencies in existing knowledge and have explained how they are going to address the gap, then they are well on the way to suggesting why the work is needed. Sometimes, they may have already discussed why the deficiency needs to be filled. If not, then the next section involves explaining the reasons why the hole needs to be packed. A useful strategy is to identify the people who will benefit (Creswell, 2014). From a knowledge support perspective, for example, systematic reviews may provide a research agenda to help other investigators continue developing theory. A review might change the way academics in the discipline think about a phenomenon. From a decision support perspective, practitioners may have the evidence needed to justify actions in their professional activities. Policymakers may be able to make informed decisions. To help emphasis the review's justification, authors can identify multiple deficiencies to be addressed and audiences who will benefit.

Fifth, what is your question?   The goal of the final section in an introduction is to detail the review's purpose, plan, and propositions. Competent writers will have a sentence that explicitly states the review's purpose statement. Use phrases such as "the purpose of this review is …," "we aimed to examine …," and "the primary review goals were to …." Also, a brief overview of the review plan signposts to readers what they will learn in the following section (the method) and helps them to see the project's coherency. The method overview may include the variables or constructs under examination, the type of review (e.g., meta-analysis, economic evaluation, and meta-ethnography), the context, and the other aspects discussed in the previous chapter on writing purpose statements. Propositions refer to hypotheses. If suitable, hypotheses are also mentioned in the final section. Hypotheses detail reviewers' expected outcomes and are tested in a quantitative binary fashion (accepted or rejected). They may be useful when the findings are able to evaluate such dichotomous statements, such as in a meta-analysis where the significance of effects sizes can be determined. Often hypotheses are not relevant or needed, such as when a review's focus is on theory development. Hypotheses are tied to significance testing, a practice with serious limitations. Despite the ubiquity of significance testing, there have been calls for it to be abandoned, because it hinders scientific advancement (Cumming, 2012). If reviewers are going to use significance testing they would also be advised to report confidence intervals, effect sizes, and other information that helps them to interpret the meaningfulness of their findings (APA, 2010).

One useful litmus test for an introduction is to ask a colleague to read a draft version minus the purpose statement and guess the review's objectives. If the colleague can guess with some accuracy, the writer can be confident the introduction is sufficient to the task. Being able to predict the purpose suggests the introduction is written in a way that presents the review as a logical step in research activity. The final section will also provide a transition from the past research to the current review and show how the findings will rest on the shoulders of giants, perhaps a fitting metaphor because reviewers need to place themselves high enough so they can survey the landscape.

Other considerations when writing introductions include formatting, writing quality, and length. There is also the need to tailor the introduction to the audience. For example, when external stakeholders fund reviews to assist with decision-making support, they may be less interested in how projects extend current knowledge and more focused on how the outputs will help them with their needs. When producing reviews as part of postgraduate qualifications, students may have lengthy introductions to help show their understanding of the broader discipline and the research process. These considerations apply to the whole document and not just introductions.

Chapter Case Example: Are Brief Physical Activity Interventions Cost-Effective?

The review examined in this chapter is an economic evaluation of brief interventions to raise physical activity in primary care or community settings (Vijay, Wilson, Suhrcke, Hardeman, & Sutton, 2016). The article has open access so you can freely download it from the *British Journal of Sports Medicine*'s website (volume 50,

pages 408–417). Broadly, the introduction conforms to Kendall et al.'s (2000) three act structure: it starts by positioning the research area within a broader context, it then summarizes existing knowledge, and it finishes with the review's purpose. Here, I examine the structure through the lens of the deficiencies model (Creswell, 2014). The page

numbers for direct quotes are from the electronic open access version.

First, what is being studied?
The start of the introduction focuses on the consequences of physical inactivity. The authors highlight inactivity's dire health consequences (p. 1): "physical inactivity

leads to an increased risk of developing over 20 health conditions, including coronary heart disease (CHD), cancer, type two diabetes and stroke." Further, these consequences cost substantial amounts of money. The tension is then broken with hope: physical activity is good for health. The opening finishes by revealing that despite efforts having been made to promote physical activity and the knowledge that it is healthy, only 39% of men and 29% of women get sufficient levels.

Second, what is already known?

The next stanza summarizes existing knowledge in a logical fashion. The authors highlight that there exist a number of interventions known to increase physical activity and have national guidelines to support their use (we learn later the evidence comes from meta-analyses and systematic reviews). Despite political interest in implementing these interventions, the limited financial resources force funders to ensure that cost-effective strategies are rolled out, one type of which are brief interventions. Here the introduction transitions into the next section.

Third, what is unknown?

The authors identify a deficiency in knowledge about the cost-effectiveness of brief physical activity interventions. Although economic evaluation reviews exist they have been broad in scope ("these reviews evaluated the cost-effectiveness of physical activity in general," p. 2) and are outdated. Further, the authors write: "the lack of economic evidence for brief interventions in physical activity has been recognised" (p. 2). From this point, it is likely that readers will be able to guess the review's purpose.

Fourth, who will benefit?

There is no separate section on the benefits of conducting the review that follows on from the identification of the gap. Instead, the authors move straight to the purpose statement. In this review, the introduction is short, consisting of six paragraphs and less than 600 words. Previously, the authors had discussed how understanding the cost-effectiveness of physical activity interventions would help policymakers reach decisions about which ones to implement. Given the brevity of the introduction, restating

the benefits may have led to redundant repetition. Although Creswell's (2014) deficiency model helps writers to fashion logical well-structured introductions, the framework is best viewed as good advice rather than a necessity.

Fifth, what is the question?

The final sentence in the introduction details the review purpose (p. 2): "we tailored our search to a specific question, that is, 'What do we currently know about the cost-effectiveness of brief interventions delivered in primary care or community settings to increase physical activity?'" The question contains several of the components of good quantitative review questions discussed in ▶ Chapter 2. The authors (a) signal the purpose statement, (b) identify the variables and present them in a logical order that indicates how they might relate to each other, and (c) mention the research setting. The reader has a clear understanding of the project's purpose and what they might read about in the remainder of the article.

Summary

Alfred Korzybski (1933), the semanticist, wrote "a map is not the territory it represents, but, if correct, it has a similar structure to the territory, which accounts for its usefulness" (p. 58). Although introductions are maps, they are written for specific purposes: to justify the review being presented. Authors who develop introductions that faithfully represent the knowledge terrain will find it easier to identify the holes and sections that need landscaping. Identifying the ways in which a review will advance knowledge provides one avenue by which to justify the project. A second avenue focuses on decision support or impact. In what ways will beautification of the knowledge terrain allow people to make decisions about policy, interventions, resource allocation, or how to live? Introductions that demonstrate how a review provides knowledge and decision-making support set the stage for projects that readers will find engaging and be interested in learning about. The current chapter has provided guidance on how to structure introductions that lead to well-justified review questions. Authors who are working from sufficiently detailed and accurate maps can begin building their review methods with confidence. In the next chapter, I start to focus on method construction by focusing on inclusion and exclusion criteria which set the scope or the boundaries of the evidence on which the review's findings will be based.

❷ Learning Exercises

1. Locate two systematic reviews and ask a friend to blank out their purpose statements. Then read the introductions and write out the reviews' likely objectives in your own words. Uncover the reviews' actual published aims and compare them to the ones you wrote.
   - Ask yourself which of the purpose statements seem more coherent with the introductions: the ones you wrote or the published aims.
   - If you had difficulty identifying the purpose statements, evaluate what changes are needed to the introductions to better foreshadow the reviews' objectives.
2. Locate another review, ideally in the area of your interest, and delete or cover up the introduction. Read the remainder of the document. You may, if you wish, read the review's purpose statement if located in the final introductory paragraph. Now sketch out an introduction according to either Creswell's (2014) or Kendall et al.'s (2000) frameworks.
3. You could undertake exercise 2 in parallel with a friend who is focused on a different review. Swap the introductions each of you have written, leaving out the purpose statements. Try to recreate the review objectives based on the introductions each of you has written. Provide each other with feedback on the strengths and limitations of your work.
4. Start developing your introduction: After completing the learning exercises in Chapters 1–3, you will now have an initial draft of the protocol with a detailed purpose statement. Either revisit or add an introduction and evaluate if it mirrors Creswell's (2014) deficiency model or not. Ask yourself if the introduction has:

- Cast an opening lure that identifies the content area in an engaging manner to hook the reader's interest.
- Presented a clear and critical picture of current knowledge.
- Revealed the ways that the review will advance knowledge.
- Shown how the review might assist knowledge support.
- A purpose statement containing the features outlined in ▶ Chapter 3.

References

APA. (2010). *Publication manual of the American Psychological Association* (6th ed.). Washington, DC: Author.

Bem, D. J. (2004). Writing the empirical journal article. In J. M. Darley, M. P. Zanna, & H. L. Roediger III (Eds.), *The compleat academic: A career guide* (2nd ed., pp. 185–219). Washington, DC: American Psychological Association.

Booth, A., Sutton, A., & Papaioannou, D. (2016). *Systematic approaches to a successful literature review* (2nd ed.). Thousand Oaks, CA: Sage.

Borenstein, M., Hedges, L. V., Higgins, J. P. T., & Rothstein, H. R. (2009). *Introduction to meta-analysis.* Chichester, UK: Wiley.

Chalmers, I., Hedges, L. V., & Cooper, H. (2002). A brief history of research synthesis. *Evaluation and the Health Professions, 25,* 12–37. ▶ https://doi.org/10.1177/0163278702025001003.

Creswell, J. W. (2014). *Research design: Qualitative, quantitative, and mixed methods approaches* (4th ed.). Thousand Oaks, CA: Sage.

Cumming, G. (2012). *Understanding the new statistics: Effect sizes, confidence intervals, and meta-analysis.* New York, NY: Routledge.

Gough, D., & Thomas, J. (2017). Commonality and diversity in reviews. In D. Gough, S. Oliver, & J. Thomas (Eds.), *An introduction to systematic reviews* (2nd ed., pp. 43–70). Thousand Oakes, CA: Sage.

Kendall, P. C., Silk, J. S., & Chu, B. C. (2000). Introducing your research report: Writing the introduction. In R. J. Sternberg (Ed.), *Guide to publishing in psychology journals* (pp. 41–57). Cambridge, UK: Cambridge University Press.

Korzybski, A. (1933). *Science and sanity: An introduction to non-Aristotelian systems and general semantics.* Englewood, NJ: Institute of General Semantics.

Murayama, K., & Elliot, A. J. (2012). The competition-performance relation: A meta-analytic review and test of the opposing processes model of competition and performance. *Psychological Bulletin, 138,* 1035–1070. ▶ https://doi.org/10.1037/a0028324.

Pawson, R., Greenhalgh, T., Harvey, G., & Walshe, K. (2004). *Realist synthesis: An introduction.* Manchester, UK: Economic and Social Research Council.

Smith, M. L., & Glass, G. V. (1977). Meta-analysis of psychotherapy outcome studies. *American Psychologist, 32,* 752–760. ▶ https://doi.org/10.1037//0003-066X.32.9.752.

Thomas, J., O'Mara-Eves, A., Harden, A., & Newman, M. (2017). Synthesis methods for combining and configuring textual or mixed methods data. In D. Gough, S. Oliver, & J. Thomas (Eds.), *An introduction to systematic reviews* (2nd ed., pp. 181–209). Thousand Oaks: Sage.

Tod, D., Edwards, C., & Cranswick, I. (2016). Muscle dysmorphia: Current insights. *Psychology Research and Behavior Management, 9,* 179–188. ▶ https://doi.org/10.2147/PRBM.S97404.

Vijay, G. C., Wilson, E. C. F., Suhrcke, M., Hardeman, W., & Sutton, S. (2016). Are brief interventions to increase physical activity cost-effective? A systematic review. *British Journal of Sports Medicine, 50,* 408–417. ▶ https://doi.org/10.1136/bjsports-2015-094655.

Inclusion and Exclusion Criteria

© The Author(s) 2019
D. Tod, *Conducting Systematic Reviews in Sport, Exercise, and Physical Activity*,
https://doi.org/10.1007/978-3-030-12263-8_5

Learning Objectives

After reading this chapter, you should be able to:
- Explain the value of unambiguous inclusion and exclusion criteria.
- Write clear inclusion and exclusion criteria.
- Use inclusion and exclusion criteria to identify relevant studies.

Introduction

A cadastral surveyor's principal role is to establish property boundaries. Drawing on maps, records, legal documents, and physical land surveys, these professionals locate and mark a property's boundaries. The advantage to landowners is the clear division between their estates and those belonging to other people. Owners can then use their land knowing they are within the limits of their properties. Similarly, systematic reviewers need to identify the boundaries of the evidence landscape they propose to survey and distinguish it from the terrain in which they lack interest. Reviewers do not use physical boundary markers, but a conceptual equivalent: inclusion and exclusion criteria. Ideally, these yardsticks are established prior to the formal search and define the types of evidence being sought. In reviews with multiple iterations and searches, inclusion and exclusion criteria might change throughout the project's lifecycle. The criteria used for each individual search, however, are established before the literature hunt begins.

The quality of the land markers in cadastral surveying may not influence the establishment of boundaries. Any object unlikely to move over time will suffice. In systematic reviews, however, inclusion and exclusion criteria have a substantial influence on the project. For example, vague, incomplete, or uninterpretable criteria make it difficult for investigators to decide whether or not to accept or reject the studies located. Irrelevant criteria send reviewers in wrong directions. Individuals who develop specific, relevant, and interpretable criteria will make conducting and reading reviews easier for themselves, colleagues, editors, stakeholders, and other consumers. In this chapter, I focus on inclusion and exclusion criteria, explain their benefits, provide guidelines on their construction, and illustrate their use.

The Value of Unambiguous Inclusion and Exclusion Criteria

Unambiguous inclusion and exclusion criteria operationally define the review question (Card, 2012). Operational definitions detail the key characteristics of constructs in concrete terms. To illustrate, the operational definition of VO_2 max could be an individual's final result on a maximal oxygen uptake test. The operational definition of a ground reaction force could be the number measured by a force platform. The operational definition of competitive anxiety could be the score people achieve on a competitive anxiety questionnaire. In systematic reviewing, inclusion and exclusion criteria define the types of evidence suitable to answering the question. For example, some of the inclusion and exclusion criteria suitable for reviews examining relationships between exercise frequency and appearance satisfaction might stipulate that studies should have (a) measured the number of days per week individuals exercised, (b) recorded participants' scores on a validated appearance satisfaction inventory, and (c) calculated a correlation coefficient. Inclusion and exclusion criteria are extensions of a review's purpose, and help investigators describe the specific components in their objectives (e.g., participants, variables, outcomes, etc.).

Inclusion and exclusion criteria also contribute to transparency, a key systematic review value (Petticrew & Roberts, 2006). Transparency allows readers to evaluate the adequacy of inclusion and exclusion criteria, and in principle, helps them to find the same studies if they repeated the search. Achieving transparency requires thought, because there is much variation by which primary studies are undertaken, reported, labelled, and indexed.

Sometimes, inclusion and exclusion criteria need explanation and justification (Card, 2012). For example, the criteria that studies need to have evaluated coach education programmes may appear straightforward. Coach education programmes, however, vary according to content, delivery strategy, time investment, assessment, underpinning pedagogical theory, etc. Clear criteria help to reduce unwanted heterogeneity among studies. Poorly defined inclusion and exclusion criteria risk reviewers comparing apples with oranges, bananas, and even kiwifruit.

Unambiguous criteria reduce subjectivity in the search and selection of literature (Petticrew & Roberts, 2006). The influence of ambiguous criteria is not reduced by having experienced reviewers undertake the search. Experience is not related to decision-making accuracy or consistency in systematic reviews (Horton et al., 2010). Difficulties in accepting or rejecting studies may reflect suboptimal inclusion and exclusion benchmarks. Reduced subjectivity allows enhanced consistency, both within a person and across individuals. Criteria can also help to evaluate decision shift or wobble: the degree to which reviewers' application of the criteria has varied over time. Inclusion criteria assist in maximizing intra and interpersonal reliability.

Writing Clear Inclusion and Exclusion Criteria

Criteria ideally follow from the purpose statement. Typically in sport, exercise, and physical activity, inclusion and exclusion criteria focus on (a) primary research design (what type of method is suitable for answering the question?), (b) conduct (was the method implemented correctly?), and (c) relevance (does the data provide helpful information? Treadwell, Singh, Talati, McPheeters, & Reston, 2011). The ease in which reviewers can develop inclusion and exclusion criteria may be one indicator of their review question's adequacy. Just as mnemonics, such as PICO and SPIDER, help individuals clarify review questions, these tools can also guide the development of suitable inclusion and exclusion criteria.

To illustrate using PICO, reviewers may ask: "in volleyball players, does the combination of plyometric sessions plus normal training, compared with usual training, lead to increased vertical jump height?" Possible inclusion criteria may help target studies that have:

— Sampled volleyball players (*Participants*).
— Included individuals who undertook usual training plus plyometric sessions (*Intervention*).
— Assessed participants who completed only their normal training (*Comparison*).
— Measured vertical jump height as a dependent variable (*Outcomes*).

In this example, reviewers might transform PICO into PICOR, where R represents research design, to ensure they focus on experimental research so they can assume causality when interpreting results.

Research design Reviewers sometimes consider two issues regarding research design: primary research quality and type (Meline, 2006). Regarding quality, as discussed previously, critical appraisal is a feature of well-conducted reviews. Numerous scoresheets and tools exist to help individuals with critical appraisal (see ▶ Chapter 8). These tools may sometimes be integrated with the inclusion and exclusion criteria, but doing so needs justification. For example, some critical appraisal tools are designed to generate numerical scores reflecting a study's quality (a contested practice, see ▶ Chapter 8), and reviewers might exclude studies totalling below a threshold, because they desire to base findings on the highest quality evidence available. The practice, however, may eliminate sound studies that were poorly written up, especially older ones published before reporting standards existed. Before eliminating studies, reviewers could ask the primary research authors to provide additional information if available. Deleting studies also prevents authors from examining how methodological features influence results (Card, 2012).

More broadly, there is debate over the suitable breadth of inclusion criteria regarding primary research quality (Meline, 2006). Some people suggest a broad approach is ideal and reviewers should consider studies regardless of quality. An alternative view is that reviewers should only synthesize studies meeting some high methodological standard of rigour. A broad approach risks an *over-inclusion threat* (Meline), where synthesis is difficult or meaningless, because of study heterogeneity. A narrow view risks an *over-exclusion threat* (Meline) that limits the clinical application or generalizability of the review findings. Abrami, Cohen, and d'Apollonia (1988) offered a compromise in which authors describe in detail their criteria and reasons for excluding individual studies. Further, reviewers can also analyse primary research strengths and weaknesses, with these results contributing to knowledge.

Regarding study type, particularly in health-related fields, primary research is often discussed in the shadow of the methodological hierarchy of evidence (Walach & Loef, 2015). The hierarchy ranks evidence according to the method that generates it, such as placing expert opinion at the bottom and meta-analytic reviews of randomized controlled trials at the apex. Reliance on the hierarchy privileges numerical experimental research over other ways of examining the world (Andersen, 2005). The hierarchy is a useful tool when used in the right context, such as research focused on evaluating intervention effectiveness or the examination of causal relationships. The hierarchy is less useful in other contexts, such as when investigators undertake qualitative research to explore the ways people interpret and make sense of their lives. Slavish devotion to the hierarchy carries the (sometimes erroneous) implication that certain types of research (e.g., qualitative inquiry) are inferior to other forms of investigation (e.g., randomized controlled trials).

There have been acrimonious debates regarding research design over the years in sport, exercise, and physical activity research communities, with the most notable being the mud-slinging associated with the quantitative and qualitative divide. Much of this debate has missed a key point: researchers should identify the best method for answering the question under investigation (Sackett & Wennberg, 1997), a principle applicable to reviews as well as primary research. Selecting research conducted with suitable methods helps ensure a meaningful synthesis.

Participants Describing the type of participants primary researchers need to have examined helps to assess the generalizability or transferability of a review's results (Meline, 2006). A non-exhaustive list of possible characteristics includes gender, age, ethnicity, sexual orientation, personality attributes, geographical region, or medical condition. The final characteristics used ideally mirror the review purpose and theoretical orientation. Tod and Edwards (2015), for example, focused on males in their meta-analysis of the relationship between the drive for muscularity and exercise-related behaviour, arguing that gender moderated how people interpreted muscularity and existing measures were suitable for males only. Finally, some characteristics are self-explanatory (e.g., age in years), whereas others need description (e.g., child or adult).

Intervention, exposure, or phenomena A challenge in some sport, exercise, and physical activity research areas is finding studies where interventions or phenomena of interest are sufficiently similar to allow meaningful groupings to occur. Interventions, for example, vary in their duration, number of sessions, delivery mode, etc. Contextual settings vary in personnel, culture, management style, etc. Reviewers have to decide how to group studies, sometimes on the basis of insufficient details. Narrowing the criteria may increase study homogeneity, but may also reduce the number of eligible studies and generalizability of findings. A compromise is to follow-up a main analysis with a moderator assessment. For example, if a review examines the influence of nutritional supplementation on a performance measure, then a moderator analysis might focus on dosage levels.

Comparison Researchers either compare the results from one group with another (between-participants design) or from one sample who experienced two or more conditions (within-participant design). Not all control groups or conditions are equal. For example, when examining the effect of self-talk on sport skill execution, researchers have used *no-instruction, do your best, placebo, distraction* or other control groups or conditions (Hardy, Oliver, & Tod, 2009). It may be unclear if these conditions are equivalent. Reviewers need to demonstrate that different control groups can be combined in the one analysis, or perhaps run a moderator or sensitivity assessment.

Sometimes in sport, exercise, and physical activity research, the term *control group* may be unsuitable. The American Psychological Association, for example, has suggested that the term control group be applied cautiously if researchers have not fully randomized samples or controlled confounding variables that could modify outcomes (Wilkinson & Task Force on Statistical Inference, 1999). Instead, the term *contrast group* may be suitable. To illustrate, participants in self-talk research who are assigned to a *do your best* control condition may spontaneously engage in self-talk. The comparison in these studies is not between a self-talk intervention and a non-self-talk control group. Instead, the comparison is between people who were asked to engage in self-talk and individuals asked to do their best, which is a different question.

Outcomes   Opinions vary about whether outcomes should, or should not, be used as inclusion or exclusion criteria (Meline, 2006). The resolution depends on factors, such as the review's purpose, focus, underlying theory, stakeholders, intended audiences, and profile of included outcomes. For example, if the research question is "what are the social implications of promoting leisure tourism in previously under-developed areas?" it would be advisable that outcomes are avoided as inclusion and exclusion criteria unless the authors are confident that they know all the social implications that might fall within the question's domain. If the question, however, is "what are the effects of leisure tourism on employment rates in underdeveloped areas?" then employment rate measures may be an inclusion criterion.

Sometimes a review question might lead to a large number of outcomes being included in the project. For example, a review question focused on the correlates of doping is broad and likely to generate a long list of variables. Researchers would probably need to draw on theory to help them interpret the meaningfulness of the findings. In some cases, it may help to differentiate between primary, secondary, and trivial outcomes (c.f., O'Connor, Green, & Higgins, 2011). Primary outcomes are necessary for substantial knowledge advancement or decision-making purposes. Secondary outcomes may be useful, but less helpful than primary variables. Trivial outcomes contribute little to knowledge or decision support.

A related issue refers to variable calibration and meaningfulness. Indirect, analogue, or surrogate variables are common in the sport, exercise, and physical activity research. In the social science sub-disciplines, for example, variables are often assessed using questionnaires, but it is typically unclear what the scores from these measures mean in terms of real world metrics (Andersen, McCullagh, & Wilson, 2007). For example, on an exercise motivation question, what does a difference of 2 units in a 6-point Likert scale mean in terms of behaviour? Will people scoring 3 on the inventory exercise more days a week than individuals scoring 2? If so, how many more days a week? The answers are typically unknown. Stakeholders may not care about questionnaire scores, but want to know the real world implications of the research findings.

Other possible inclusion criteria   The list of possible inclusion and exclusion criteria is long and the characteristics invoked are determined by various factors, such as the review question and logistical considerations. Examples of additional criteria include publication language, year, country of origin, or type. Criteria imposed for logistical reasons may be necessary to allow a review to be completed, but limit the findings' generalizability or lead to biased results. Country of origin is one example. Reviewers may focus on research conducted in Western settings or even in one specific country. Findings from these reviews may not transfer to non-Western contexts, or even other Western countries. Sound reasons may exist for limiting reviews to Western-based studies, but authors need to justify them and then reflect on the implications in their discussions.

Creating and Using Inclusion and Exclusion Criteria

Step 1: Developing and testing criteria   Developing the inclusion and exclusion criteria may involve an iterative process of refinement during review conceptualization and construction (see ► Chapter 2). During conceptualization, criteria may be adjusted as reviewers scope the likely literature base, consult stakeholders, and explore what questions may be feasible or relevant. Initial criteria flexibility, however, varies across projects. In some reviews, such as those aggregating results quantitatively, the criteria may be relatively easy to develop if the variables and components can be defined in straightforward ways. For other projects, the activities of scoping the literature, developing the question, and modifying criteria may occur over several iterations. In some cyclical approaches to synthesizing literature (e.g., realist syntheses), the iterations may occur throughout the project's life, during which inclusion and exclusion criteria may change depending on the targeted studies.

Such adjustments do not permit teams to make up and change inclusion and exclusion criteria on a whim. Instead, often these cycles can be anticipated and built into the protocol, with any refinement being documented. To illustrate, investigators reviewing literature on applied sport and exercise psychologist development might adopt an iterative approach that echoes a realist synthesis type method. Initially, the researchers might identify a relevant theory describing practitioner professional growth and propose two waves of searching and synthesis. The first wave might focus on sport psychology literature to compare context-specific evidence for the professional development theory being evaluated. Specific clear inclusion and exclusion criteria would be developed and tailored to the objectives of the first wave. After completing wave one, the investigators may identify gaps in the evidence and use these to focus a second search on coaching, clinical, education, and counselling psychology literature to ascertain what might be learned from related disciplines. New inclusion and exclusion criteria will be developed for the second wave of searching. Ideally, these separate waves would be described in the review protocol, but the inclusion and exclusion criteria for the second search may need adjustment and documentation.

Assessing reliability across reviewers helps teams evaluate the adequacy of their inclusion and exclusion criteria. Calculating agreement metrics, such as Cohen's kappa or Bangdiwala's B (Munoz & Bangdiwala, 1997), helps teams decide if criteria are specific, relevant, complete, and interpretable. Low agreement metrics may emerge from reviewer mistakes or inconsistent primary research reporting (Centre for Reviews and Dissemination, 2009; Meline, 2006). Disagreements are likely to occur, and when developing their protocols, reviewers benefit from establishing methods to resolve differences.

Step 2: Using the criteria   When searching for literature, study selection typically starts with a title and abstract review of each article. Studies clearly meeting at least one of the exclusion criteria are rejected (Centre for Reviews and Dissemination, 2009; Meline, 2006). During the title and abstract review, authors normally retain papers where it is unclear if the study meets the selection criteria. A final decision is deferred until the full-text assessment, to prevent eligible articles being rejected.

The full text is obtained for articles remaining after the title and abstract search. During full-text assessment, reviewers decide if the study (a) satisfies each inclusion criteria, and (b) does not fulfil any exclusion benchmarks. It is good practice to document reasons why articles have been rejected at the full-text assessment stage, and involve two people making the decision independently of each other. Rejection and reliability information can then be reported in review outputs. Item 17, for example, of the PRISMA standards of reporting stipulates that reviewers provide the number of studies screened, assessed for eligibility, included in the review, and excluded (with reasons) at each stage.

Two obstacles that may emerge during full-text assessment include a lack of information on which to make final decisions and the processing of large numbers of papers. First, when there is a lack of information, reviewers may approach the primary researchers. These individuals may not reply, or if they do, may not have the information requested. Reviewers then reject the study because of insufficient information. Second, although some methodologists argue each paper should be assessed independently by at least two people, such a stipulation represents an ideal that may not be realistic if a broad search was conducted. Instead, samples of each reviewer's assessments may be checked by an independent person.

During study selection, reviewers need to be sensitive to multiple reports from the same study (Centre for Reviews and Dissemination, 2009). Duplication may occur because researchers have published their work in different languages, reported different outcomes across papers, employed different data analysis procedures, or published the same study with an increased sample size. Primary researchers do not always acknowledge multiple papers from the same study and it may not be easy to identify when it has occurred. Contacting authors helps to avoid double counting of results (Borenstein, Hedges, Higgins, & Rothstein, 2009).

Chapter Case Example: How Can Sport Contribute to Positive Youth Development?

The purpose in Holt et al.'s (2017) recent project was to create a model of positive youth development through sport by reviewing qualitative literature. The article appeared in the *International Review of Sport and Exercise Psychology*, Vol. 10, pages 1–49, although open access versions may be freely downloaded from various websites. The two specific objectives included: (a) reviewing and evaluating qualitative studies of sport-related positive youth development, and

(b) analysing and synthesizing these studies' findings. Investigations were included if they:

- Reported primary data obtained using at least one qualitative data collection technique (e.g., interview, observation).
- Had been conducted with participants in organized and adult-supervised competitive sport, recreational sport, or other settings that included sport activities.
- Had made specific reference to positive youth development in the title or purpose statement, or used positive youth development research in some way.

To help define these criteria, the authors stated that (a) mixed methods studies were included if qualitative data could be separated and examined independently from quantitative data, and (b) investigations of life skills were included, because they fit in the overall positive youth development umbrella. Studies excluded included:

- Literature reviews, methodological papers, conceptual/ theoretical papers, conference abstracts, theses/dissertations, government/ nongovernmental documents, and non-profit organization reports, because they did

not contain original data or had not been subject to peer review.
- Articles that examined health or positive outcomes in the absence of a positive youth development perspective.

SPIDER is one tool to guide inclusion and exclusion criteria in reviews of qualitative research (Cooke, Smith, & Booth, 2012). SPIDER stands for Sample, Phenomenon of interest, Design, Evaluation, and Research type. Applying SPIDER to Holt et al. (2017) reveals that studies were included if investigators had:

- S: sampled participants in settings that included organized and adult-supervised competitive, recreational, or other sport activities
- Pi: focused on positive youth development in organized sporting activities
- D: used at least one qualitative data collection technique
- E: examined features of positive youth development
- R: employed either a qualitative or mixed-method research type.

Holt et al. excluded unpublished reports, or those documents produced outside of normal scientific publishing channels, and often labelled *grey literature* (Benzies, Premji, Hayden, & Serrett, 2006), because "they

either did not contain original data or had not been subjected to peer review." Publication bias may occur if rejecting documents on the basis that they were not peer reviewed. For example, theses or non-profit organization reports may have contained relevant data, but were dismissed because they were not peer reviewed. Peer review, however, may well have been undertaken, but not reported. In Commonwealth countries, for instance, Ph.D. dissertations are typically reviewed by two or three markers, and can be considered to have received some version of peer review. Further, the fact that an article was peer reviewed is not a guarantee of quality given the known problems with the process (Bruce, Chauvin, Trinquart, Ravaud, & Boutron, 2016). As mentioned above, one key feature of systematic reviews is the evaluation of the quality of available evidence. Grey and non-peer reviewed literature can still be assessed against the same quality control criteria as published studies.

In a second example, Roig et al. (2009) compared eccentric with concentric training on muscle strength and mass gains. From a PICO perspective, included investigations had:

- P: samples of healthy adults aged 18-65 years
- I: eccentric training programmes

- C: concentric training programmes
- O: measured muscle strength, muscle mass, or both.

Also, studies had to be randomized controlled trials or clinical controlled trials, and full text had to be available. Roig et al. excluded investigations that:

- Had not been randomized controlled trials or clinical controlled trials.
- Had sampled participants with any pathology.

- Had not compared eccentric and concentric training.
- Had assessed training programmes not meeting the minimum duration or frequency requirements.
- Had not measured either muscle strength or mass.
- Had washout periods of 1 month or less following training with alternate muscle actions or contralateral limbs.
- Had not been written in English.

It is common for reviews to exclude non-English language papers. Many review teams do not have members able to translate relevant articles written in languages other than English or have translation funds. Such inability introduces potential bias to the review. Research written in languages other than English may have relevant data to help to provide an answer with greater depth, breadth, or precision than the result obtained.

Summary

Many sports, games, and physical activities are played within clearly defined areas marked by flags, white lines, fences, or other means. These markers help keep events manageable, feasible, and meaningful. Without markers, the games and sports may be unplayable if participants become so spread out they cannot interact. Similarly, systematic review inclusion and exclusion criteria help project teams stay within the boundaries of their knowledge field. Well-crafted criteria are broad enough to ensure that the necessary relevant evidence is captured, but narrow enough to help keep reviews manageable. One way they help keep projects feasible is by influencing the development of search terms or keywords. The construction of search strategies is the focus of the next chapter.

❓ Learning Exercises

1. Locate two systematic reviews in an area of your choice. This exercise may be especially effective with two reviews on the same question. On a sheet of paper draw a table with three columns, headed up "question," "inclusion and exclusion," and "search strategy." Write out the relevant information from both reviews under each heading. Consider the following questions:
   - Is there coherency across the three columns; that is, do the inclusion and exclusion criteria follow logically from the question? Does the search strategy reflect the criteria?
   - Evaluate if you think there is an optimal balance between breadth and narrowness of inclusion and exclusion criteria.
   - What changes, additions, or deletions would you make to the criteria to produce a better fit with the question and search strategy?

2. Open up a textbook in your major discipline (e.g., sports journalism) and select two variables that you believe may be related (e.g., "athlete gender" and "newspaper coverage"). Using these two variables:
   - Develop a question that could guide a systematic review (e.g., does newspaper sports coverage differ by athlete gender?) that also conforms to the guidelines in ▶ Chapter 3.
   - With the question in mind, develop suitable inclusion and exclusion criteria that conform to either the PICO or SPIDER acronym.
   - Give your question and criteria to a friend, ask them to detail any changes they might make, and discuss any differences.
3. Review the inclusion and exclusion criteria listed in the review protocol you developed in ▶ Chapter 2. You may find it helpful to use a table similar to the one in the first exercise to guide your thinking.

References

Abrami, P. C., Cohen, P. A., & d'Apollonia, S. (1988). Implementation problems in meta-analysis. *Review of Educational Research, 58*, 151–179. ▶ https://doi.org/10.3102/00346543058002151.

Andersen, M. B. (2005). Coming full circle: From practice to research. In M. B. Andersen (Ed.), *Sport psychology in practice* (pp. 287–298). Champaign, IL: Human Kinetics.

Andersen, M. B., McCullagh, P., & Wilson, G. J. (2007). But what do the numbers really tell us? Arbitrary metrics and effect size reporting in sport psychology research. *Journal of Sport and Exercise Psychology, 29*, 664–672. ▶ https://doi.org/10.1123/jsep.29.5.664.

Benzies, K. M., Premji, S., Hayden, K. A., & Serrett, K. (2006). State-of-the-evidence reviews: Advantages and challenges of including grey literature. *Worldviews on Evidence-Based Nursing, 3*, 55–61. ▶ https://doi.org/10.1111/j.1741-6787.2006.00051.x.

Borenstein, M., Hedges, L. V., Higgins, J. P. T., & Rothstein, H. R. (2009). *Introduction to meta-analysis.* Chichester, UK: Wiley.

Bruce, R., Chauvin, A., Trinquart, L., Ravaud, P., & Boutron, I. (2016). Impact of interventions to improve the quality of peer review of biomedical journals: A systematic review and meta-analysis. *BMC Medicine, 14*, article 85. ▶ https://doi.org/10.1186/s12916-016-0631-5.

Card, N. A. (2012). *Applied meta-analysis for social science research.* New York, NY: Guilford.

Centre for Reviews and Dissemination. (2009). *Systematic reviews: CRD's guidance for undertaking reviews in health care.* York, UK: Author.

Cooke, A., Smith, D., & Booth, A. (2012). Beyond PICO: The SPIDER tool for qualitative evidence synthesis. *Qualitative Health Research, 22*, 1435–1443. ▶ https://doi.org/10.1177/1049732312452938.

Hardy, J., Oliver, E., & Tod, D. (2009). A framework for the study and application of self-talk within sport. In S. D. Mellalieu & S. Hanton (Eds.), *Advances in applied sport psychology: A review* (pp. 37–74). London, UK: Routledge.

Holt, N. L., Neely, K. C., Slater, L. G., Camiré, M., Côté, J., Fraser-Thomas, J., ... Tamminen, K. A. (2017). A grounded theory of positive youth development through sport based on results from a qualitative meta-study. *International Review of Sport and Exercise Psychology, 10*, 1–49. ▶ https://doi.org/10.1080/1750984X.2016.1180704.

Horton, J., Vandermeer, B., Hartling, L., Tjosvold, L., Klassen, T. P., & Buscemi, N. (2010). Systematic review data extraction: Cross-sectional study showed that experience did not increase accuracy. *Journal of Clinical Epidemiology, 63*, 289–298. ▶ https://doi.org/10.1016/j.jclinepi.2009.04.007.

Meline, T. (2006). Selecting studies for systematic review: Inclusion and exclusion criteria. *Contemporary Issues in Communication Science and Disorders, 33*, 21–27.

Munoz, S. R., & Bangdiwala, S. I. (1997). Interpretation of Kappa and B statistics measures of agreement. *Journal of Applied Statistics, 24*, 105–112. ▶ https://doi.org/10.1080/02664769723918.

O'Connor, D., Green, S., & Higgins, J. P. T. (2011). Defining the review question and developing criteria for including studies. In J. P. T. Higgins & S. Green (Eds.), *Cochrane handbook for systematic reviews of interventions*. Version 5.1.0 [updated September 2011]: The Cochrane Collaboration. Retrieved from ► www.cochrane-handbook.org.

Petticrew, M., & Roberts, H. (2006). *Systematic reviews in the social sciences: A practical guide*. Malden, MA: Blackwell.

Roig, M., O'Brien, K., Kirk, G., Murray, R., McKinnon, P., Shadgan, B., & Reid, W. D. (2009). The effects of eccentric versus concentric resistance training on muscle strength and mass in healthy adults: A systematic review with meta-analysis. *British Journal of Sports Medicine, 43*, 556–568. ► https://doi.org/10.1136/bjsm.2008.051417.

Sackett, D. L., & Wennberg, J. E. (1997). Choosing the best research design for each question. *British Medical Journal, 315*, 1636. ► https://doi.org/10.1136/bmj.315.7123.1636.

Tod, D., & Edwards, C. (2015). A meta-analysis of the drive for muscularity's relationships with exercise behaviour, disordered eating, supplement consumption, and exercise dependence. *International Review of Sport and Exercise Psychology, 8*, 185–203. ► https://doi.org/10.1080/1750984X.2015.1052089.

Treadwell, J. R., Singh, S., Talati, R., McPheeters, M. L., & Reston, J. T. (2011). *A framework for "best evidence" approaches in systematic reviews*. Plymouth Meeting, PA: ECRI Institute Evidence-based Practice Center.

Walach, H., & Loef, M. (2015). Using a matrix-analytical approach to synthesizing evidence solved incompatibility problem in the hierarchy of evidence. *Journal of Clinical Epidemiology, 68*, 1251–1260. ► https://doi.org/10.1016/j.jclinepi.2015.03.027.

Wilkinson, L., & Task Force on Statistical Inference. (1999). Statistical methods in psychology journals: Guidelines and explanations. *American Psychologist, 54*, 594–604. ► https://doi.org/10.1037/0003-066x.54.8.594.

Undertaking Search Strategies

© The Author(s) 2019
D. Tod, *Conducting Systematic Reviews in Sport, Exercise, and Physical Activity*,
https://doi.org/10.1007/978-3-030-12263-8_6

Learning Objectives

After reading this chapter, you should be able to:
— Translate review questions into suitable search keywords.
— Undertake electronic and non-electronic searches.
— Identify suitable information sources and databases.
— Develop effective search strategies.
— Present search results according to recognized standards.

Introduction

Are systematic reviews original research? People disagree in their answers to this question. For example, whereas 70% of medical journal editors agree, 30% do not (Meerpohl, Herrle, Antes, & von Elm, 2012). Although academics may vary in their opinions, drawing parallels between primary research and systematic reviews is helpful for understanding the synthesis process. Sampling frame is one example (Card, 2012). In primary research, investigators accept that surveying whole populations is typically unrealistic and they work with samples instead. The principle also applies to the review process. Although a population of studies exists to answer a review question, it is normally unrealistic to expect authors to locate them all. The population is ever growing, often ill-defined, greatly dispersed, and littered with investigations not readily available.

One challenge in the review process is the identification of suitable studies, and even with electronic databases and moves to make research and datasets freely available, searching is typically one of the most time-consuming aspects of a review and has been described as "remarkably difficult" (Chalmers, Dickersin, & Chalmers, 1992). Despite the challenges, there are ways to manage the search so reviewers can be confident they have sufficient evidence to yield meaningful answers to their questions. In this chapter, I discuss the process and issues associated with literature searching.

A guiding aim is to maximize sensitivity (or recall) and specificity (or precision) (Petticrew & Roberts, 2006). A sensitive search finds the relevant studies and a specific search avoids locating irrelevant studies. The two ideas share an inverse relationship. Highly sensitive searches typically have low specificity (i.e., they return a lot of irrelevant studies) because the strategy involves widening the net (Petticrew & Roberts, 2006). Highly specific searches might return a lower number of records to examine, but carry an increased risk of missing relevant studies. Given the variation in research design, keywords, indexing, and methodological reporting in the sport, exercise, and physical activity domains, scholars may accept low specificity to ensure high sensitivity.

Phases in the Literature Search

❑ Figure 6.1 presents the search phases, that include scoping, electronic searches, manual searches (or citation chasing), verification, and documentation (Booth, Sutton, & Papaioannou, 2016). During aggregative reviews, the scoping search normally occurs

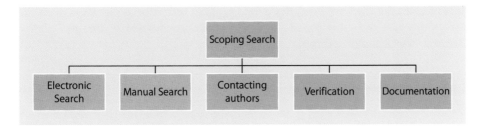

◻ Fig. 6.1 Phases involved in a literature search

in the construction phase and the formal search during the conduct phase. The litera-ture search may be less linear and more cyclical in configurative reviews. Further, the activities might be conducted in a parallel rather than serial fashion.

Scoping Search

Scoping reviews "aim to map *rapidly* the key concepts underpinning a research area and the main sources and types of evidence available" (Mays, Roberts, & Popay, 2001, p. 194). The scoping review helps to assess the value of, and plan for, a full system-atic review, although they may be discrete projects with their own products (Arksey & O'Malley, 2005). As a preliminary search, scoping exercises involve estimating the primary research quantity and quality, based on a small number of databases, existing reviews, and other sources (Booth et al., 2016). The outcomes may include:

- Refining the review questions and scope.
- Selecting databases and other information sources.
- Establishing key search terms.
- Creating search strategies tailored to the electronic databases to be employed.
- Allowing researchers to develop, pilot, and document their overall search plan (Long, 2014).

An overall search plan is a description of the various avenues investigators will travel along to locate literature. Regarding keywords, reviewers may begin by analysing sem-inal papers to generate search terms, a technique known as pearl growing (Booth et al., 2016). Thesauri also help to flesh out the search terms. Keywords can then be arranged according to the review question to develop a generic search strategy.

To illustrate, consider the question: "in non-adult males (*participants*), what effect does motivational self-talk (*intervention*), compared with instructional self-talk (*com-parison*) have on muscular force development (*outcome*)?" Example keywords might be arranged as:

- *Participants*: child, teenager, male, men, young adult, adolescent, boy.
- *Intervention*: motivational self-talk, positive self-talk, inner dialogue, self-talk.
- *Comparison*: instructional self-talk, technical self-talk.
- *Outcome*: muscular force, strength, endurance, power, weight/resistance training.

Investigators can then use Boolean operators, along with database thesauri (if available), to translate the above generic keyword framework into search strategies tailored to individual electronic archives.

Formal Search

The formal search involves implementing strategies reviewers identified from the scoping exercise. As presented in ◘ Fig. 6.1, there are various ways to locate relevant studies including: electronic archives, citation chasing or manual searching, and author contact. The strategies are not mandatory, but rather investigators can select how, and to what extent, they use them to achieve their review goals. For example, in sport, exercise, and physical activity the preponderance of evidence most often occurs in scientific journals, books, and monographs. The highest yield strategies include searching electronic archives and citation chasing, with author contact being of lesser value.

Electronic Search

Electronic databases are a staple of modern systematic reviews, and are typically the first or primary tool investigators employ. Despite being the search backbone, being able to drive a database effectively is a skill requiring coaching and practice. The variation across the numerous electronic databases is one reason their use is not straightforward. ◘ Table 6.1 provides examples of databases investigators in sport, exercise, and physical activity may employ. Consulting a librarian or information scientist is a

◘ Table 6.1   Example electronic databases
SPORTDiscus
Web of Science
ABI/INFORM Collection
Annual Reviews
CINAHL
Pubmed
Cochrane library
ERIC
MEDLINE
ProQuest
PsycARTICLES
PsycINFO
Scopus
EThOS

useful tactic when first climbing into the driver's seat. Two considerations include coverage and search strategy translation (Booth et al., 2016; Brunton, Stansfield, Caird, & Thomas, 2017).

Database coverage   Reading the descriptive documentation accompanying electronic databases provides insight into their coverage and helps reviewers decide which ones to use. They vary in the features included. Some databases index grey literature, conference presentations, books, magazines, and theses as well as journal articles. Depending on user access level, full-text may be included. Databases also vary in the breadth of coverage. For example, well-established and high impact journals from the dominant publishers are more likely to be indexed than younger, less-established, or predator journals. The number of years back databases cover also fluctuates. Searching multiple databases is desirable given the variation across them (Bramer, Giustini, Kramer, & Anderson, 2013).

Electronic databases also differ in the ancillary functions they provide to enhance the search experience. For example, some databases provide the located study's reference list, articles that have cited the located article, or both. These functions assist with citation chasing (see below). In addition to the citation details and abstracts, databases may also supply other useful information. To illustrate, PubMed suggests similar articles that may be of interest. Scopus provides metrics detailing a citation's influence and community engagement (e.g., revealing how the number of citations for an article compares against the average for similar outputs).

Tailoring search strategies   Given database variation, tailored search strategies are more effective than generic versions. Various functions assist tailoring, including thesauri, Boolean and other operators, field limits, and search filters. It is beyond the scope of this book to describe the details of individual databases. Instead, I focus on providing overall guidance. The information below might be easier to comprehend with an example search strategy. ► Box 6.1 presents a strategy Liu and Latham (2009) designed for the Cochrane library database and used in their review of resistance training's effects on physical function in older adults. Search strategies across databases look different because of different symbols and available features. Standardization of operators, thesauri, and limits is not complete, increasing the difficulty for one person to be a jack of all databases. Reviews published in the Cochrane library include their search strategies for each database, and it is helpful to read these to become familiar with their development.

Box 6.1: Liu and Latham's (2009) Cochrane library database search strategy
#1 ((strength* or resist* or weight*) NEAR/3 training):ti,ab,kw
#2 (progressive resist*):ti,ab,kw
#3 #1 OR #2
#4 MeSH descriptor Exercise, this term only
#5 MeSH descriptor Exercise Therapy, this term only
#6 (exercise*):ti,ab,kw

#7 (#4 OR #5 OR #6)
#8 (resist* or strength*):ti,ab,kw
#9 (#7 AND #8)
#10 (#3 OR #9)
#11 (elderly or senior*):ti,ab,kw
#12 (#10 AND #11)

Database *thesauri* or *controlled vocabularies* are lists of keywords, typically presented in a hierarchal fashion, to assist with indexing consistency and searching. Thesauri allow reviewers to employ the same keywords indexers assign to records. The hierarchical listing of keywords helps reviewers to broaden and narrow their searches to balance recall with precision (sensitivity with specificity). Medical Subject Headings (MeSH) is an example thesaurus used in various databases such as PubMed. ▶ Box 6.2 gives an example of how terms are listed within MeSH. Although helpful, the concepts that reviewers are interested in are not always in thesauri and investigators may need to combine thesaurus terms with free text keywords in their searches (Booth et al., 2016). Also, the words reviewers use to describe a concept may not be the same as those in the thesauri.

Box 6.2: Example fragment from the MeSH thesaurus
Human Activities [I03]
- ▬ Leisure Activities [I03.450]
  - – Recreation [I03.450.642]
    - – Camping [I03.450.642.159]
    - – Dancing [I03.450.642.287]
    - – Gardening [I03.450.642.378]
    - – Hobbies [I03.450.642.469]
    - – Play and Playthings [I03.450.642.693]
    - – Sports [I03.450.642.845]
      - – Athletic Performance [I03.450.642.845.054]
      - – Cardiorespiratory Fitness [I03.450.642.845.054.300]
      - – Physical Endurance [I03.450.642.845.054.600]
      - – Physical Fitness [I03.450.642.845.054.800]
        - – Cardiorespiratory Fitness [I03.450.642.845.054.800.500]
      - – Baseball [I03.450.642.845.110]
      - – Basketball [I03.450.642.845.117]
      - – ....

Keywords can be combined using *Boolean logic* to expand or narrow searches to enhance recall and precision. Boolean commands include AND, NOT, and OR.
- ▬ OR expands searches: "sport OR exercise" will retrieve articles with either term.
- ▬ AND narrows searches: "sport AND exercise" will retrieve articles with both terms.

- NOT narrows searches: "sport NOT exercise" will retrieve articles with the term "sport" if they do not include the term "exercise".

As well as Boolean operators, databases also offer features to overcome limitations with spelling, synonyms, and alternative keyword phrasing. *Wildcard* symbols can be used to include various spelling and related words. In SPORTDiscus, the "?" and "#" symbols are wildcards. When "?" is used, searches return all words with a letter in the space: "m?n" will find records with either "men" or "man." If "#" is included, searches find all citations with the word that appears with or without the extra character; for example, "colo#r" finds citations containing "color" or "colour." In SPORT-Discus, "*" is used for *truncation*. For example, "comput*" returns records containing "compute," "computer," or "computing." "A midsummer's * dream" will return results containing "a midsummer's night dream".

Continuing in SPORTDiscus, when users enclose a phrase in double quotation marks (e.g., "sports medicine") the search engine returns records with the exact phrase. *Proximity* searches locate records with two or more words occurring within an identified number of words of each other. Proximity operators consist of a letter (N or W) and a number and are placed between the search words. For example, "N4" returns records with the words if they are within four words of one another regardless of order. "Drive N4 muscularity" will search for "muscularity drive" and "drive for muscularity." "W4" finds the words if they are within four words of one another and in the specified order. "Drive W4 muscularity" will search for "drive for muscularity" but not "muscularity drive." Multiple terms can be used on either side of the operator: "(baseball OR football OR basketball) N5 (teams OR players)" will search for "baseball teams," "baseball players," "football teams," "football players," "basketball teams," and "basketball players."

Search filters are strategies written to retrieve particular records in a database, such as those of a specific research design (e.g., qualitative), document type (e.g., review), or focus of interest (e.g., quality of life). Filters tend to be tailored towards specific databases, because search rules are not standardized across archives. Although they can assist reviewers in locating relevant studies, filters are best used with caution and when investigators can find evidence for their effectiveness. For example, McKibbon, Wilczynski, and Haynes (2006) designed and tested filters for locating qualitative studies in PsychINFO. Search filters of interest to sport, exercise, and physical activity researchers can be found at:

- King's College London (▶ http://libguides.kcl.ac.uk/systematicreview/SRFilters).
- Scottish Intercollegiate Guidelines Network (SIGN; ▶ http://www.sign.ac.uk/search-filters.html).
- Cochrane online handbook, section 6.4.11 (▶ http://training.cochrane.org/handbook)
- McMasters University (▶ https://hiru.mcmaster.ca/hiru/HIRU_Hedges_MEDLINE_Strategies.aspx).
- The InterTASC Information Specialists' Sub-Group Search Filter Resource (▶ https://sites.google.com/a/york.ac.uk/issg-search-filters-resource/home).

Searches can also be restricted by imposing *search limits*. In SPORTDiscus, for example, the search limits include full-text availability, publication year, language, and thesaurus term. Keywords can also be restricted to specific fields. As with search strategies, considering the limits available helps to prevent reviewers from biasing their projects. For example, restricting a search to journal articles may result in publication bias. As another example, some databases (e.g., Scopus) allow reviewers to search by author name. Although searching by author may be helpful if prolific individuals exist in the area, it may add bias to the search and constrain the breadth of critical thought (Booth et al., 2016).

Electronic databases are powerful in the hands of knowledgeable and experienced reviewers. Even in the hands of an expert, however, one database is insufficient for most projects. To improve the effectiveness of their efforts, reviewers can develop and compare more than one strategy for a database, use multiple electronic archives, employ manual search strategies, and include a librarian or information scientist in the team.

Grey Literature

Grey or fugitive literature refers to work outside the normal scientific publishing channels (Benzies, Premji, Hayden, & Serrett, 2006; Petticrew & Roberts, 2006). Examples of grey literature include unpublished studies, occasional papers, and informal publications. Theses and conference proceedings might also be classed as grey literature, although these documents may be listed in electronic databases, such as Web of Science and ProQuest. Grey literature is produced by various groups, including universities, charities, local and central government, commercial and public organizations, research funders and councils, sporting bodies, and health organizations. Databases exist to help reviewers locate grey literature and examples include:

- Open DOAR (▶ http://www.opendoar.org/).
- Grey Matters (▶ https://www.cadth.ca/resources/finding-evidence/grey-matters).
- The Grey Literature Report (no longer being updated; ▶ http://www.greylit.org/home).
- OpenGrey (▶ http://www.opengrey.eu/).
- Social Care Online (▶ https://www.scie-socialcareonline.org.uk/).
- PsycEXTRA (▶ http://www.apa.org/pubs/databases/psycextra/index.aspx).
- Open Access Theses and Dissertations (OATD; ▶ https://oatd.org/).
- Networked Digital Library of Theses and Dissertations (NDLTD; ▶ http://search.ndltd.org/).

A search of grey literature helps to alleviate publication bias. Given that grey literature is outside normal delivery channels, reviewers can never know if they have obtained all, most, or even a representative sample. One value of networking with colleagues and stakeholders is that they can help point reviewers to likely sources of fugitive work.

Citation Chasing or Manual Searching

Electronic database searches will likely miss relevant studies (McManus et al., 1998), and are best complemented with additional citation chasing strategies. One common technique is a *backward search* where investigators scan the reference lists of located articles. Scanning reference lists helps reviewers identify historical studies, going back to the seminal papers in the area. Relevant studies, however, that have not been widely cited may be missed.

Some databases, such as Google Scholar and Scopus, allow *forward searching* in which the papers citing a located study may be identified. Forward searching is limited by publication lag time and the frequency with which databases are updated. These limitations may be relevant in popular and fast-moving areas of science. The speed at which science moves is one reason why the Cochrane Collaboration suggests reports are produced within three months of the search and reviews are updated every two years (Green & Higgins, 2011).

Another strategy is a journal or book table of contents search. In some sport, exercise, and physical activity disciplines, however, studies may not emerge in a table of contents or database searches, because authors have not provided clear titles and keywords reflecting their work. Some authors, for example, may have pithy or otherwise ambiguous titles preventing easy indexing or search return likelihood. To illustrate, although cute, the title "The long and winding road" (Tod, 2007) does not contain any terms relevant to a search on sport psychologist professional development which was the focus of the article. Table of contents searches are labour intensive, with potentially lower yields per time investment than other strategies. Reviewers need to assess the cost–benefit ratio in deciding how much emphasis to give the method (Booth et al., 2016).

Contacting Authors

Contacting researchers has several benefits before, during, and after a search. Prior to a search, colleagues can provide feedback on a protocol that may lead to an improved method. During a search, they can provide additional unpublished articles. After a search, colleagues can comment on the adequacy of the process and database.

Also, if located articles are missing information, then colleagues can supply details to keep the studies in the review. In some sport and exercise research areas, considerable numbers of studies risk being excluded from systematic reviews, because they do not contain information relevant to the project. For example, studies are frequently excluded from meta-analyses because authors have not provided basic information, such as descriptive statistics or correlations. This risk is especially associated with older studies produced before current publication standards started emerging, although even current authors frequently do not write complete reports for various reasons (e.g., word limits or page restrictions).

The number of primary research authors that reviewers approach varies from all of them to just the most active in the field. The decision is based on time, resources, and need. When contacting authors I have found the following to be helpful:

- Explain the review's purpose.

— Identify the specific studies I seek (provide citation details) or the criteria detailing what studies I desire.
— Detail the information needed for study inclusion (e.g., effect sizes).
— Outline what I will do with the information.
— State I will cite their work and give appropriate credit.
— Indicate I am willing to analyse their data myself if they cannot provide the details.
— Outline I will not share their data with others and will delete it from my computer once I gathered the information needed for my project.

Response rates vary with projects. It is not always possible to locate authors' contact details, especially with older studies where authors have retired from academia or are no longer publishing. Many times the first author was a student at the time of the study and is no longer engaged in research. In such cases, contacting second or subsequent authors may allow requested information to be secured. Frequently, authors who do respond are unable to provide assistance because they did not keep their raw data or other information (a common occurrence with conference presentations that have not been published). An increasing number of organizations, journals, and universities are making studies, supplementary information, and raw data freely available on the internet as a result of calls for researchers to be transparent and accountable for their work. Such movements are helpful for systematic reviewers. Finally, although reviewers may make use of social media, professional networking sites, forums, and blogs, I have found contacting individuals directly on a personal basis yields greater help.

Search Verification

The purpose of verification is to assess the quality of the search (Booth et al., 2016): has it been adequate? In primary research, investigators typically attempt to demonstrate the rigour of their work. For example, quantitative researchers discuss ideas such as validity and reliability. If systematic reviews are a type of research, then quality control is a relevant component (see ▸ Chapter 10). Regarding the literature search, process and outcome are two quality control yardsticks: has the search been undertaken in a suitable manner and did it locate the relevant evidence? Reviewers who demonstrate they have upheld the values underpinning systematic synthesis will build confidence in readers and stakeholders.

Reviewers can assess the quality of their search via consultation with other experts including researchers, consumers, information scientists, and librarians (Brunton et al., 2017). Evaluation can start early in the process. For example, experts can comment on the protocol to help establish if the process is likely to be adequate. Consultation can occur throughout the search and experts can offer perspectives on issues that arise or when reviewers are unsure about some aspect. After a search has finished an expert can conduct an audit trail to assess if the process was sound. Consultation may allow reviewers to have confidence in their search process, but not the outcome, because the expert's assessment is reliant on recall ability and knowledge of the research.

Another strategy is for two individuals to perform the search independently of each other and then compare notes and results. Such an approach speaks to the reliability of a search, not its validity. High agreement among the two individuals reveals that the search was performed consistently, but does not show that it was adequate to the task. Nevertheless, reliability is a necessary, but insufficient, component of validity. A well-planned search is inadequate if performed haphazardly. Having two people perform the search independently can be a time-consuming endeavour and maybe be infeasible. An alternative is for one person to conduct the search and a second individual to perform a sample of the activities throughout the process. The two reviewers then compare and discuss their results. For example, the second person may perform backward and forward searches on 20% of the located studies.

A third possible strategy is for investigators to crosscheck their results with previous reviews identified prior to the search and which have not been subject to backward or forward citation chases. Although the strategy may have face validity, it is limited to the date at which earlier reviews were produced and also does not account for publication lag time. Despite these limitations, it is a useful strategy for suggesting that historically relevant papers have been surveyed.

If the verification process unearths additional papers, then investigators need to identify the reasons why the documents were missed (Card, 2012). For example, are the documents actually indexed in the electronic databases employed? Were their keywords different from those used in the search? Identifying why papers were missed may provide insights that help reviewers modify and improve their search (Brunton et al., 2017).

Search Documentations

A desirable principle to follow when documenting a search is to provide enough detail so the process is replicable. The replication principle ensures reviewers uphold two key systematic review values: transparency and reproducibility. If sufficiently detailed, people replicating a search will likely return similar numbers of studies, although results are unlikely to be exactly the same for various reasons, such as new research having been reported or database search engines having been modified.

There are two aspects to document: search processes and outcomes (Booth et al., 2016; Brunton et al., 2017). To help illustrate, ◨ Table 6.2 presents relevant items from the PRISMA checklist that indicate the type of information reviewers benefit from recording (Moher, Liberati, Tetzlaff, Altman, & The Prisma Group, 2009). Regarding the process, useful information includes the inclusion/exclusion criteria, databases searched, years of coverage, date of last search, electronic and manual search strategies with limits and filters, contact with authors, study selection process, and verification efforts. Regarding search outcomes, most systematic review reporting standards stipulate that investigators present the number of papers identified, excluded, and retained at each phase of the search. The PRISMA flowchart is a common way to present search results and is freely available on the web (▶ http://prisma-statement.org/prismastatement/flowdiagram.aspx; Moher et al., 2009). Maintaining a version of the diagram throughout the search is one method to assist documentation of outcomes.

A range of reporting standards and associated checklists exist to assist reviewers when documenting and presenting their searches. These standards are sometimes tailored towards specific types of reviews. The PRISMA checklist, for example, addresses

□ Table 6.2   Items from PRISMA checklist related to search documentation

Topic	Item #	Item description
Eligibility criteria	6	Specify study characteristics (e.g., PICOS, length of follow-up) and report characteristics (e.g., years considered, language, publication status) used as criteria for eligibility, giving rationale
Information sources	7	Describe all information sources (e.g., databases with dates of coverage, contact with study authors to identify additional studies) in the search and date last searched
Search	8	Present full electronic search strategy for at least one database, including any limits used, such that it could be repeated
Study selection	9	State the process for selecting studies (i.e., screening, eligibility, included in systematic review, and, if applicable, included in the meta-analysis)
Study selection	17	Give numbers of studies screened, assessed for eligibility, and included in the review, with reasons for exclusions at each stage, ideally with a flow diagram

all aspects of a systematic review and is focused on randomized controlled trials. STARLITE is another example that was developed for qualitative research (Booth, 2006). STARLITE stands for:

— **S**ampling strategy
— **T**ype of study
— **A**pproaches
— **R**ange of years
— **L**imits
— **I**nclusion and exclusions
— **T**erms used
— **E**lectronic sources.

Other examples are listed at the systematic review toolbox website (▶ http://systematic-reviewtools.com/index.php), a user-driven catalogue of tools that support the systematic review process.

When to Stop Searching

There are no rules about when to stop a search, and investigators are usually uncertain about how complete their efforts have been, because the population of relevant studies is almost always unknown (Petticrew & Roberts, 2006). A number of guidelines have been proposed, including statistical estimation of coverage, stakeholder satisfaction, and comparison against some standard, although limited evidence exists for them (Booth, 2010). For configurative reviews, theoretical saturation may be a reasonable guideline, whereby reviewers search until additional relevant studies fail to provide evidence that modifies the synthesis findings (Petticrew & Roberts, 2006). In aggregative reviews, investigators need to take into account the project's purpose, time constraints, available resources, reviewer energy, stakeholder needs, and search yields when they make decisions about when to stop. The ideal exhaustive search, whereby all possible sources are tapped using the broadest and most sensitive search strategies until the returns reach zero, is generally not feasible (Brunton et al., 2017). Instead, individuals will demonstrate the quality of their search by showing that they have made all reasonable efforts to locate relevant studies, and have estimated the likely number and effect of the missing works (Petticrew & Roberts, 2006).

Document Management

For systematic reviews on sport, exercise, or physical activity topics, the end result of a search is a collection of studies or other documents that satisfy the inclusion and exclusion criteria and form the foundation on which the synthesis findings will rest. The collection of papers may range from a few (perhaps as low as zero) to hundreds. Engaging in some form of methodical document management will help reviewers keep track of studies, so the energy expended in locating papers results in a high-quality product. Various options exist ranging from the use of index cards to software that helps manage the entire systematic review process, such as SUMARI from the Joanna Briggs Institute. Options in between the two extremes include generic spreadsheet or database software (e.g., Microsoft Excel or Access) and reference management packages (e.g., Paperpile, Endnote, or Mendeley). The documents themselves might be printed and stored in a filing cabinet or kept electronically on computers. The choice about the document management system employed is influenced by the number of studies returned from the search, the reviewers' preferences and expertise, and needs of the project. The greater the sophistication and scope of the project, the more the use of specialist software may yield benefits. Teams using specialist software, however, need to ensure they have people with the expertise to drive the technology. For example, meta-analytic reviews of large numbers of primary studies may benefit from tailored systematic review software such as RevMan (Cochrane Collaboration) or EPPI-Reviewer 4 (Evidence for Policy and Practice Information-Centre). Alternatively, index cards and filing cabinets may be adequate for small scale reviews. As well as searching for reporting standards and tools at the systematic review toolbox discussed above, investigators can learn about possible document management software options, including both free and commercial packages.

Chapter Case Example: Psychological Terms Used in Youth Talent Development

The example in the current chapter is Dohme, Backhouse, Piggott, and Morgan's (2017) review of the psychological terms used in youth talent development literature. The article was published in the *International Review of Sport and Exercise Psychology, Vol. 10*, pages 134–163. Authors' pre-published versions are available through Google Scholar.

Purpose

The three core aims were:

(1) to identify the terms used that describe the psychological components perceived to facilitate the development of talented athletes to elite performers; (2) to locate and analyse the definitions and descriptions of the terms used in order to identify consistencies and inconsistencies; (3) to group, label and, define any clustered psychological terms. (p. 138)

Scoping review

A scoping review was undertaken in which the authors created and trialled keywords using SPORTDiscus. Every tenth result was evaluated for relevance and additional keywords. The procedures were repeated until the authors believed they had identified the most effective search terms. The final list included: "('psychological characteristic*' OR 'mental skill*' OR 'psychological skill*' OR 'mindset') AND (elite OR success* OR excellen* OR perform*) AND develop* AND (young OR athlet*) NOT disorder" (p. 139). The use of a scoping review to identify a list of keywords is a strong positive feature of the current example, because the authors demonstrated an evidence-based approach to the creation of their search method.

Inclusion criteria

The inclusion criteria included:

(1) peer-reviewed research studies;

(2) published in English language only; (3) published between January 2002 (when the first relevant study in relation to the research purpose could be identified) and May 2015 (when the formal search was finalised); (4) have gathered original qualitative or quantitative evidence on psychological components that facilitate young (under 18 years of age) talented athletes' development; (5) involve sporting activities as defined by the Oxford Dictionary of Sport Science and Medicine (Kent, 2006); (6) contain specific reference to either psychological/ mental characteristics, psychological/mental skills, psychological/mental qualities, psychological/ mental attributes, psychological/mental techniques, psychological/ mental factors, psychosocial characteristics, mindset, or life skills within the title or abstract; and (7) include data compatible and relevant to the three core aims of this study. (p. 139)

Similar comments made in the last chapter about using peer-review and language status as inclusion criteria are relevant for the current example and reflect possible sources of publication bias. The authors made attempts to justify and define the inclusion criteria, a feature not always present in reviews in sport, exercise, and physical activity. Their justifications reflect a commitment to ensuring transparency in the review.

Formal search

The databases searched included SPORTDiscus, PsycINFO, PsycARTICLES, and ERIC. The authors also engaged in backward searching. The authors may have considered a forward search and a journal table of contents search, but the use of multiple databases and a backward search were strong features.

Documentation and verification

The investigators presented a full PRISMA diagram and all the information requested in the PRISMA checklist as detailed in ▣ Table 6.2. Regarding verification, the authors state that the reference list from their search "was examined by an experienced external advisory team. Suggestions from this advisory team regarding additional references were considered and 12 papers accessed and reviewed; following this process, an additional 3 references were added" (p. 139). Having independent experts pass judgement on the reference list was an unusual but positive feature of the project because most reviews in our disciplines do not undertake the method. As an addition, it would have been useful if the authors had presented their reflections on the feedback. For example, did they consider any modifications to their search given that the experts suggested three additional papers?

Summary

A satisfying milestone in primary research is often the completion of data collection. The completion of a literature search may be not quite as pleasing in a systematic review because science does not stop. Researchers continue "relentlessly hewing away at the coalface of science" (Petticrew & Roberts, 2006, p. 99), churning out new studies. Reviewers may need to rerun and update their searches before their projects are complete. It is difficult to update a search efficiently if it has been conducted in an arbitrary, slapdash, or disorganized manner. Instead, a well-planned and implemented search, that has been sufficiently documented, allows investigators to minimize the time and effort needed to scan the knowledge base for the most recent work. In this chapter, I have discussed ways to build and undertake search strategies that will help form a solid foundation for the next feature in the review process: data extraction, the topic of the following chapter.

❓ Learning Exercises

1. Identify two electronic databases you might use in your own research. Visit the Cochrane library (▶ http://onlinelibrary.wiley.com/cochranelibrary/search) and locate two or three reviews relevant to your topic. Turn to the appendices containing the search strategies and examine those listed for your chosen databases. You may need to access the databases and open their help pages. Can you:
   - Explain each of the various symbols and abbreviations?
   - Follow the flow of the search strategy?
   - Identify any redundancy in the strategy?
   - See any potential gaps?
2. Exercise 2 in ▶ Chapter 5 asked you to develop a review question along with inclusion and exclusion criteria. Using the results from that exercise:
   - Develop search terms you could use to locate literature.
   - To complement these you could also read two or three seminal papers in the area to help source additional keywords (pearl growing).
   - Select two databases and construct possible tailored search strategies.
   - Implement the search strategies and if you have access to relevant software, download the results into the package, record the numbers, and delete duplicates.
   - Reflect on the process and use your thoughts to help you with exercise 3.
3. Review the search strategy you created for the protocol you wrote during ▶ Chapter 2. Modify it in light of the current chapter and the above exercise. In particular:
   - Detail any scoping activities you think need to be undertaken.
   - Select the various for search methods that you think are relevant to your topic.
   - Develop a plan for documenting and verifying the quality of the search.

References

Arksey, H., & O'Malley, L. (2005). Scoping studies: Towards a methodological framework. *International Journal of Social Research Methodology, 8,* 19–32. ► https://doi.org/10.1080/1364557032000119616.

Benzies, K. M., Premji, S., Hayden, K. A., & Serrett, K. (2006). State-of-the-evidence reviews: Advantages and challenges of including grey literature. *Worldviews on Evidence-Based Nursing, 3,* 55–61. ► https://doi.org/10.1111/j.1741-6787.2006.00051.x.

Booth, A. (2006). "Brimful of STARLITE": Toward standards for reporting literature searches. *Journal of the Medical Library Association, 94,* 421–429.

Booth, A. (2010). How much searching is enough? Comprehensive versus optimal retrieval for technology assessments. *International Journal of Technology Assessment in Health Care, 26,* 431–435. ► https://doi.org/10.1017/S0266462310000966.

Booth, A., Sutton, A., & Papaioannou, D. (2016). *Systematic approaches to a successful literature review* (2nd ed.). Thousand Oaks, CA: Sage.

Bramer, W. M., Giustini, D., Kramer, B. M. R., & Anderson, P. F. (2013). The comparative recall of Google Scholar versus PubMed in identical searches for biomedical systematic reviews: A review of searches used in systematic reviews. *Systematic Reviews, 2,* article 115. ► https://doi.org/10.1186/2046-4053-2-115.

Brunton, G., Stansfield, C., Caird, J., & Thomas, J. (2017). Finding relevant studies. In D. Gough, S. Oliver, & J. Thomas (Eds.), *An introduction to systematic reviews* (2nd ed., pp. 93–122). Thousand Oaks, CA: Sage.

Card, N. A. (2012). *Applied meta-analysis for social science research.* New York, NY: Guilford.

Chalmers, I., Dickersin, K., & Chalmers, T. C. (1992). Getting to grips with Archie Cochrane's agenda. *British Medical Journal, 305,* 786–788. ► https://doi.org/10.1136/bmj.305.6857.786.

Dohme, L. C., Backhouse, S., Piggott, D., & Morgan, G. (2017). Categorising and defining popular psychological terms used within the youth athlete talent development literature: A systematic review. *International Review of Sport and Exercise Psychology, 10,* 134–163. ► https://doi.org/10.1080/1750984X.2016.1185451.

Green, S., & Higgins, J. P. T. (2011). Preparing a Cochrane review. In J. P. T. Higgins & S. Green (Eds.), *Cochrane handbook for systematic reviews of interventions.* Version 5.1.0: Cochrane Collaboration. Retrieved from ► www.cochrane-handbook.org.

Liu, C. J., & Latham, N. K. (2009). Progressive resistance strength training for improving physical function in older adults. *Cochrane Database of Systematic Reviews,* article CD002759. ► https://doi.org/10.1002/14651858.cd002759.pub2.

Long, L. (2014). Routine piloting in systematic reviews—A modified approach? *Systematic Reviews, 3,* article 77. ► https://doi.org/10.1186/2046-4053-3-77.

Mays, N., Roberts, E., & Popay, J. (2001). Synthesising research evidence. In N. Fulop, P. Allen, A. Clarke, & N. Black (Eds.), *Studying the organisation and delivery of health services: Research methods* (pp. 188–220). London, UK: Routledge.

McKibbon, K. A., Wilczynski, N. L., & Haynes, R. B. (2006). Developing optimal search strategies for retrieving qualitative studies in PsycINFO. *Evaluation & the Health Professions, 29,* 440–454. ► https://doi.org/10.1177/0163278706293400.

McManus, R. J., Wilson, S., Delaney, B. C., Fitzmaurice, D. A., Hyde, C. J., Tobias, R. S., ... Hobbs, F. D. R. (1998). Review of the usefulness of contacting other experts when conducting a literature search for systematic reviews. *British Medical Journal, 317,* 1562–1563. ► https://doi.org/10.1136/bmj.317.7172.1562.

Meerpohl, J. J., Herrle, F., Antes, G., & von Elm, E. (2012). Scientific value of systematic reviews: Survey of editors of core clinical journals. *PloS One, 7,* article 35732. ► https://doi.org/10.1371/annotation/b9a9cb87-3d96-47e4-a073-a7e97a19f47c.

Moher, D., Liberati, A., Tetzlaff, J., Altman, D. G., & The Prisma Group. (2009). Preferred reporting items for systematic reviews and meta-analyses: The PRISMA statement. *PLoS Medicine, 6,* article 1000097. ► https://doi.org/10.1371/journal.pmed.1000097.

Petticrew, M., & Roberts, H. (2006). *Systematic reviews in the social sciences: A practical guide.* Malden, MA: Blackwell.

Tod, D. (2007). The long and winding road: Professional development in sport psychology. *The Sport Psychologist, 21,* 94–108. ► https://doi.org/10.1123/tsp.21.1.94.

6

Data Extraction

© The Author(s) 2019
D. Tod, *Conducting Systematic Reviews in Sport, Exercise, and Physical Activity*,
https://doi.org/10.1007/978-3-030-12263-8_7

Learning Objectives

After reading this chapter, you should be able to:
- Discuss the need for data extraction tools.
- Identify the information to extract for your own projects.
- Develop effective extraction code sheets and codebooks.
- Select from among possible extraction tools and software.
- Create evidence tables and systematic maps.

Introduction

During data extraction, reviewers read the full text of the final sample of included investigations and mine the information they will analyse, synthesize, and interpret. Along with the search, data extraction is one of the core tasks separating systematic from black box reviews (Gough, Oliver, & Thomas, 2017). Individuals often combine data extraction with critical appraisal, or the assessment of a study's quality. For clarity, however, I discuss these activities in separate chapters. Useful outcomes from data extraction include evidence tables and systematic maps, and both these products provide descriptive overviews of the reviewed studies. Extraction involves data reduction and is somewhat similar to quantitative factor analysis or qualitative thematic content analysis. Researchers aim to drain the large pools of information contained in the located studies to manageable levels to avoid drowning in data. In this chapter, I discuss the reasons for adopting a methodical approach to extraction, discuss the types of information to collect, detail how to tailor an extraction tool for a specific project, and introduce evidence tables and systematic maps as a prelude to data analysis and synthesis.

Data Extraction Purposes

Written reports of primary studies vary in many ways for different reasons, such as journal space limitations, researchers' abilities and preferences, discipline-specific norms, journal style preferences, and peer review inconsistency. The divergent ways evidence is presented makes it challenging for reviewers to analyse and synthesize a set of studies adequately once the sample gets beyond a handful of papers. Transforming the information contained in the primary studies to a common format enhances investigators' abilities to analyse, synthesize, and interpret data to answer their review questions (Gough et al., 2017). There are four chief purposes investigators hope to satisfy from extraction in the majority of systematic reviews published in the sport, exercise, and physical activity domains: (a) prepare data for analysis and synthesis, (b) describe or chart the area under scrutiny, (c) critically appraise the quality of the primary research, and (d) manage the flow of the evidence collected throughout the project (Brown, Upchurch, & Acton, 2003).

– *Prepare data for analysis and synthesis*. Prior to analysis and synthesis, systematic reviewers typically need the data to be collated and arranged in specific ways to allow the meaning and new knowledge to arise. For example, meta-analyses are performed on numerical data arranged in spreadsheets (Borenstein, Hedges, Higgins, & Rothstein, 2009). In a meta-study examining qualitative research, extracted information is stratified according to the categories of data, method, and theory to allow the synthesis to occur (Paterson, Thorne, Canam, & Jillings, 2001). For a meta-narrative, the data may be arranged chronologically to help with identifying the evolving plotlines and stories (Greenhalgh et al., 2005).

– *Describe or chart the topic under study*. Although a descriptive survey of an area might be the main outcome of some projects, typically in sport, exercise, and physical activity, the mapping exercise provides a context for the review's main findings (Gough & Thomas, 2017). Mapping refers to representing features of the primary research in either in narrative or visual forms (Miake-Lye, Hempel, Shanman, & Shekelle, 2016). For example, maps might outline methodological features of the included studies (e.g., research designs, measures, control condition, types of interventions, participant characteristics). Maps might also provide details about the theoretical underpinnings and implications of the research in an area. Methodological and theoretical surveys allow readers to interpret review findings and place them within particular contexts. For example, describing the typical research designs employed in an area will help readers decide if they can make causal inferences from the findings. As another example, if research participants in primary studies have predominantly been females, generalizing to males may be unsuitable.

– *Critically appraise the quality of the research evidence*. A strong feature of systematic reviews is the emphasis they place on examining the rigour and quality of the underpinning evidence. Assessing research rigour and quality is discussed in ▶ Chapter 8.

– *Manage the evidence flow*. Reviewers often need to keep track of large numbers of studies throughout their projects. Even if only a few investigations are retained for analysis, normally large numbers have been screened and rejected during the search. Data extraction does not begin with reading the final sample of studies. At each stage of the search, an increasing amount of information is recorded per study (Brunton, Graziosi, & Thomas, 2017). Investigators can quickly become awash in a sea of details. Most current reporting standards, for example, suggest that the number of studies screened at each stage be documented, along with reasons for rejecting investigations at the full-text stage. A sound data extraction and collating procedure ensures reviewers will have the information if needed.

What Information to Extract

Given the time and effort involved in data extraction, methodologists advise collecting only the details needed to answer the review questions and critically appraise the evidence (Higgins & Deeks, 2011). The principle, however, implies reviewers know in advance the information they need, which may be possible in some aggregative or theory-testing reviews. When undertaking configural or theory-development reviews, authors may sometimes be uncertain about what information to extract. A helpful suggestion is to identify the minimum amount and type of data from each study reviewers believe will allow the project to answer the question, but accept adjustments may be needed along the way (Gough & Thomas, 2017). If adjustments do arise, they can be documented in revised protocols to avoid accusations of biased reporting.

☐ Table 7.1 details illustrative examples of extraction items aligned with each of the four purposes discussed above, although in practice the items might move around depending on the review purpose (Booth, Sutton, & Papaioannou, 2016; Petticrew & Roberts, 2006; Salmond & Cooper, 2017). For example, items extracted for critical appraisal in one project might be used to answer content questions in other reviews. To illustrate, evidence for a measure's validity might be a small part of the critical appraisal in some projects, but be the primary focus in reviews on that specific assessment or test. Depending on the review's scope, investigators may have to extract considerable amounts of information from sizeable bodies of evidence. Some information

7

☐ **Table 7.1**   Example items for an extraction form

Data management
Identifying elements
Study and report identifier
Data extractor
Citation details
Eligibility criteria
Inclusion criteria
Exclusion criteria

Mapping exercise
Methods
Design (e.g., experimental/observational, control group/conditions, allocation)
Participants (e.g., gender, age, ethnicity, sport, socioeconomics, student/community)
Measures
Exposure/intervention
Analysis (qualitative approach, quantitative tests)

Answer a content-driven question
Results
Descriptive
Association
Inferential
Sample and effect sizes

Critical appraisal
Quality
Risk of bias
Quality of evidence
Limitations

Additional
Funding
Author interpretations

may not be straightforward to collect and involve subjective judgement. For example, reviewers may want to examine the theoretical basis underpinning a set of qualitative studies, but primary researchers do not always discuss such details explicitly, leaving reviewers to make educated estimates. Further, multiple people might be involved in extraction. For these reasons, instituting formal data extraction tools and decision-making rules promotes consistency across people and time (Chalmers & Altman, 1995). Options available include creating a tailored code sheet, using an existing standardized tool, or a combination of both possibilities. Having a guiding tool is sensible, regardless of the investigator's familiarity in conducting reviews, because experience is not related to data extraction accuracy (Horton et al., 2010).

How to Develop an Extraction Tool

On occasion, reviewers may use off the shelf extraction tools, but more likely, however, investigators will need to modify them, or create new ones, to suit their projects. Planning, piloting, and evaluating your data extraction sheets will ensure they are fit for purpose (Elamin et al., 2009). Steps involved in creating or altering tools include (Brown et al., 2003; Sutcliffe, Oliver, & Richardson, 2017):
— Developing a code sheet and codebook.
— Establishing code sheet validity.
— Pilot testing the code sheet.
— Refining the code sheet and codebook.

Developing the code sheet and codebook Developing the coding sheet involves identifying the information needed to achieve the purposes discussed above (i.e., prepare data for analysis, map the area, critical appraisal, and manage information flow). Consulting stakeholders, colleagues, and existing research, along with reviewing the project's purpose, inclusion and exclusion criteria, and keywords, can help investigators decide what items to include in their code sheets. Reviewers can also anticipate the structure and characteristics of the findings. For example, if they wish to examine methodological moderators in a quantitative synthesis, then the code sheet will include space for variables such as participant characteristics, research design, or contextual features. Reviewers' knowledge about the data analysis methods can also help them construct their code sheet and codebook. For example, knowing that theory, findings, and method each form separate components in meta-studies allows reviewers to design code sheets that will collect information for each category.

Additional resources facilitating code sheets include codebooks and question mnemonics. The codebook mirrors the code sheet in structure, providing details to explain what information is required for each item. Codebooks contribute to extraction consistency across individuals and time. Researchers can also employ the mnemonics they may have used to develop their review questions, keywords, and search strategies to design the code sheet (e.g., PICO; Booth et al., 2016) and enhance the coherence of their reviews. For example, if the review is examining the influence of a nutritional supplement on aerobic exercise performance, some of the information the code sheet might collect could include:

- *Participants*: gender, age, height, weight, sports experience, pre-test aerobic capacity.
- *Intervention*: dosage, ingestion mechanism, regime duration.
- *Control*: control conditions.
- *Outcomes*: exercise frequency, intensity, type, time, perceived effort, post-test aerobic capacity.

Establishing code sheet validity   Submitting the code sheet and codebook to a range of individuals allows for feedback to help establish that the extraction tool will facilitate the gathering of desirable data. Reviewers, for example, might give an expert panel a blank code sheet and ask them to detail the information they would expect to see with each item, along with any other material that might help project completion.

Pilot testing the code sheet   Trialling the code sheet on some of the included studies allows reviewers to assess its adequacy. It may also be feasible to analyse the pilot data to check they will answer the review questions. As part of the pilot test, reviews might ask multiple people to extract data from a subset of the included studies to help evaluate whether or not the tool enhances decision-making consistency.

Refining the code sheet and codebook   Feedback from experts and the pilot test will help researchers adjust the code sheet and codebook. The carpenter's adage of "measure twice, cut once" is useful advice when developing collection tools. Data extraction is time-consuming. Reviewers want to minimize the number of times they read individual studies. Realizing halfway through extraction that one or more items are missing from the code sheet is unpleasant because it means re-reading material already assessed.

Higgins and Deeks (2011) make the following suggestions when designing data extraction forms:

- Include ways to identify the project and the form's version number.
- Have space to record the extractor's name and additional notes, queries, and musings.
- Include separate study and report identifiers so multiple reports of the same investigation can be linked.
- Have items assessing inclusion and exclusion eligibility placed early in forms.
- Allow space for extractors to document the location of each item's answer in the study report (e.g., page and line numbers).
- Use coded responses to minimize time and allow answers such as "unclear" or "non-reported".
- Format forms to allow straightforward transfer of information to final reports, where possible.
- Collect sample sizes associated with each outcome, as well as overall numbers.

Some of Higgins and Deek's suggestions may appear obvious to experienced reviewers, such as placing the inclusion and exclusion criteria early in the form and including ways to identify the review and primary study. Sometimes, however, novice reviewers may miss things that veterans believe are obvious.

Principles Underlying Data Extraction

Attempt to Achieve Coherency

Data extraction serves the purpose of helping maintain coherence across a review's purpose, methods, and findings. Using the mnemonics discussed in this and earlier chapters (e.g., PICO, SPIDER, etc.) can enhance coherency by helping reviewers formulate questions, identify keywords, construct inclusion and exclusion criteria, and assist in designing the data extraction sheet and codebook.

Develop Meaningful Extraction Items

There is little to be gained from collecting material not useful to a project. Reviewers typically want to be as efficient as they can and minimize the time spent extracting data. Against this backdrop, investigators benefit from planning their projects to ensure extraction forms are as brief as needed to allow the review question to be answered (Petticrew & Roberts, 2006). In some projects, such as configurative reviews focused on theory development, researchers may be unsure about what details to leave out. In these cases, if there is a chance that particular pieces of information may be helpful in satisfying the project's purpose, then it may be worth the extra time needed to collect the data. As mentioned above, decisions about what to include and leave out might be facilitated through pilot testing and consulting experts (Sutcliffe et al., 2017).

Make Items Explicit, Clear, and Unambiguous

Making extraction items explicit, clear, and unambiguous contributes to consistency across people and time. Supporting an extraction form with a codebook can increase the clarity of items. Extraction is not always straightforward, even for descriptive numerical information. For example, sometimes the sample size reported in primary research may vary across the abstract, method, and results without explanation. Attending to these types of issues in the codebook can help reviewers act consistently and justify decisions.

Qualitative Research and Data Extraction

Some reviewers of qualitative research prefer to skip the extraction phase and instead work with the original documents (Booth et al., 2016). One potential limitation with extraction forms is that they separate the data from the context of the article in which they are embedded. Also, rich description is often lost because extraction typically involves data reduction. The synthesis of qualitative research is enhanced by appreciating the context within which information is located and typically involves multiple readings of source material. A further criticism is that extraction forms imply investigators have preconceptions about what information and themes are present and relevant within the primary research. These preconceptions reflect researcher bias which may prevent an authentic portrayal of the primary investigations.

In many projects examining qualitative research, some combination of direct-to-analysis and extraction procedures will facilitate optimal progress. In most projects, for instance, there will be some data needing to be extracted and collated for all or some of the purposes outlined above. Also, it is unlikely that researchers will have no expectations about possible findings or biases that may influence the project: people are not blank slates. The absence of extraction forms does not prevent researchers' biases from influencing a project. Instead, extraction forms might provide a place where reviewers can reflect on and record their interpretations of primary studies to help them uncover their biases. Further, reviewers who pilot and assess possible extraction and direct-to-analysis protocols will have confidence in whatever strategies they employ.

Create Verification Procedures

Given that extraction error rates can approach 50%, and these mistakes can influence results (Mathes, Klaßen, & Pieper, 2017), it is sensible to undertake verification procedures. When considering corroboration methods, however, there is a time/accuracy trade-off. To illustrate, although double extraction (two people independently excavating data) yields lower error rates than single extraction (one person mining data with another individual verifying results), it also takes longer and involves more work (Buscemi, Hartling, Vandermeer, Tjosvold, & Klassen, 2006). Expecting errors and disagreements among data extractors is realistic, and planning ways to resolve differences helps maintain transparency and reduce the influence of mistakes (Shokraneh & Adams, 2017). Verification procedures can also include using people from different disciplines and with separate skills (e.g., content and method experts). Measuring concordance rates helps establish confidence in the project's rigour (Higgins & Deeks, 2011), and example measures include percentage agreement, Cohen's Kappa, or Bangdiwala's B (Munoz & Bangdiwala, 1997).

Document Data Extraction

In keeping with the transparency principle underpinning systematic reviews, most reporting standards include items focused on data extraction. The PRISMA checklist, for instance, suggests reviewers should: (a) "describe methods of data extraction from reports (e.g., piloted forms, independently, in duplicate) and any processes for obtaining and confirming data from investigators," (item 10) and (b) "List and define all variables for which data were sought (e.g., PICOS, funding sources) and any assumptions and simplifications made" (item 11). The PRISMA checklist also has items associated with risk of bias, and this topic is explored in the next chapter.

Using Existing Data Recording Tools

Reviewers can select from various ways to record the data they extract from primary studies, ranging from unsophisticated paper-based forms to tailored online systematic review software (Elamin et al., 2009; Petticrew & Roberts, 2006). Each approach has advantages and disadvantages. For example, set-up and training costs are minimal with paper-based forms, although they lack versatility and require double handling of data (e.g., from primary study to paper to electronic form for analysis). The training and set-up costs are higher for tailored systematic review software, but data may not need to be handled more than once, and the package may be able to assist or help manage analysis and synthesis. For example, in reviews employing meta-analytic techniques, some software will calculate the effect sizes needed for analysis from descriptive statistics (useful given reports often do not contain desired effect sizes). For qualitative evidence, software such as NVivo can help with the management of the volume of data often involved. The factors to consider when making a decision about what data management mechanisms to employ include the following (Elamin et al., 2009):

- Amount, complexity, and characteristics of the information to be extracted.
- Number, location, and computer literacy of the project's personnel.
- Available funding.
- Project timelines.

Many systematic reviews in sport, exercise, and physical activity involve teams of researchers undertaking small to medium size unfunded projects destined for publication in academic journals. These investigators may be dispersed across a number of institutions either within or across countries. Paper-based forms are likely impractical and there are usually insufficient funds to purchase access to tailored review software requiring a license. In these cases, reviewers are likely to choose between general purpose software, such as Microsoft Excel, or freely available systematic review packages, such as the Cochrane Collaboration's Revman. Many teams will probably use a suite of software, such as packages for information extraction (e.g., Excel), reference management (e.g., Endnote), and data analysis (e.g., N-Vivo or R).

Data Extraction Outcomes: Evidence Tables and Systematic Maps

Once unearthed, data need to be collated in an orderly manner before analysis and synthesis can occur. Two tools for collating data include evidence tables and systematic maps. Description is the essence of evidence tables and systematic maps. They provide descriptive summaries of what research has been undertaken and the associated knowledge. Evidence tables and maps represent a useful landmark in the systematic review process. It is difficult to engage in synthesis and interpretation without an adequate understanding of the existing data.

An evidence table is a common, efficient, and flexible way to collate and present information (as illustrated in ◘ Table 7.2). The typical format is to assign individual studies to a separate row in the table and each column presents some dimension, such as purpose, sample, measures, design, and findings. These tables can be placed directly

7

■ **Table 7.2** Example evidence table

Study	Purpose	Participants	Measure	Design	Major findings
Tod et al. (2018)	Effect of self-talk on vertical jump	15 male (mean age = 21.0, SD = 2.0, years) and 15 females (mean age = 22.0, SD = 2.3) students	– Jump height	Within subject design, with counterbal-anced order, repeated measures, & control conditions	– Self-talk group jump height 0.45 m (SD = 0.23 m) versus no instruction control jump height 0.34 m (SD = 0.25 m); difference significant ($P < 001$)
Edwards et al. (2016)	Effect of self-talk on vertical jump	48 male rugby players (mean age = 23.2 years, SD = 3.5)	– Jump height	Within subject design, with counterbalanced order, repeated meas-ures, & control condition	– Self-talk group jump height 0.54 m (SD = 0.15 m) versus do your best control jump height 0.44 m (SD = 0.212 m); differ-ence significant ($P < 0.01$)
…	…	…	…	…	…

Note Studies are fictional examples

into the final report, or if there are a large number of primary studies being reviewed, they can be placed in an appendix or online as supplementary materials in the case of journal publications. Tables that summarize numerical data can be imported into statistical software packages to allow quantitative analysis to occur.

A systematic or evidence map represents a step beyond the evidence table. Parkhill et al. (2011, p. 157) wrote "an evidence map is an overview of a broad research field that describes the volume, nature, and characteristics of research in that field." Depending on the review's purpose, an evidence or systematic map may be a product in its own right (and published as such) or a prelude to more detailed synthesis. The label "map" is broadly understood as indicating that the descriptive summary is presented in a visual fashion (Langer, 2015). Although reviewers can present their maps using text and tables, visual methods often illustrate the information and key messages more clearly and efficiently. The visual options are large and may include bar charts, bubble plots, flow charts, logic models, etc. Another key advantage of infographics and visual representation is they can communicate information to both professional and lay individuals who may not have the knowledge to interpret technical information.

Well-constructed maps help reviewers hypothesize links among variables in the primary research, such as associations among methodological factors and results. From such information, reviewers might identify specific questions to pursue among the primary studies (Craig et al., 2017). Maps can also reveal strengths or gaps in the literature, and stimulate a primary research agenda (Parkhill et al., 2011).

Langer (2015) evaluated the effectiveness of sport-for-development interventions on health and social outcomes in Africa and illustrates one way systematic maps can be presented. In sport-for-development initiatives, sport is a medium to address social issues. Langer reviewed 36 studies, of various designs, that assessed five types of outcomes: gender empowerment, health outcomes, socio-economic development, life skills/social capital, and social cohesion/peace. The map was underpinned by a programme theory or logic model. Reviewers use logic models or programme theories to describe the processes by which they believe interventions deliver desired results, and one example is presented in ◘ Fig. 7.1. Langer's logic model began by describing the underlying theory of the interventions (labelled input) for each outcome. Sport was either the central component of the interventions, or it was an adjunct activity to the intervention's primary focus. The inputs lead to outputs, which were example projects.

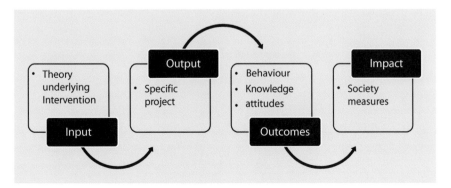

◘ **Fig. 7.1** Example logic model for Langer (2015)

The outputs influenced the outcomes, such as changes in behaviour, attitudes, and knowledge. The outcomes lead to impacts which were society wide measures. Langer showed that most of the 36 studies reviewed had focused on outcomes, and they had concentrated on changes in HIV-related knowledge, behaviour, and attitudes. No studies assessed impact (e.g., HIV infection rates) across any of the outcome types. For example, 20 studies had evaluated sport-for-development projects' effect on HIV-related knowledge ($N = 20$), HIV-related attitudes ($N = 11$), HIV-related behaviours ($N = 4$), but none on community impact, including HIV infections and prevalence ($N = 0$). Langer concluded that there was no evidence to support or refute conjectures that sport had a positive influence on health and social development in Africa, opening up a new line of inquiry.

Systematic maps typically describe rather than synthesize or interpret information. Langer's (2015) map, for example, presents the number of studies conducted dealing with each outcome, but he does not assess the findings or comment on the quality of the research. The map is supplemented with text detailing study characteristics, interventions, and outcomes to provide contextual information to assist interpretation and understanding.

Chapter Case Example: Drive for Muscularity and Health-Related Behaviour

Authors typically do not include extraction forms with publications. In the current chapter, I reflect on the extraction form and process a colleague and I used in a meta-analysis examining the relationship the drive for muscularity had with exercise behaviour, exercise dependence, disordered eating, and supplement consumption in males (Tod & Edwards, 2015). The article was published in the *International Review of Sport and Exercise Psychology*, Vol. 8, pages 185–203.

Research question

The primary purpose of the meta-analysis was to estimate the strength of the relationships that the drive for muscularity had with exercise behaviour, exercise dependence, disordered eating, and supplement use in males. One secondary purpose was to estimate the strength of the relationship between the two subscales of McCreary and Sasse's (2000) Drive for Muscularity Scale. Another secondary purpose was to assess if the relationships the drive for muscularity had with the other variables were moderated by the drive for muscularity questionnaire type, questionnaire internal reliability, and participant type (student or non-student).

Extraction datasheet constructing

We adjusted the PICO acronym to PI/ECO (Participants, Intervention/exposure, Context, and Outcome) and used it to guide the extraction sheet. The PICO acronym allowed us to map the data we needed to collect against the question we were asking. The sheet collected the following information:

- *Participants*: We recorded age, sexual orientation, ethnicity, sport participation (days/week), weight training (days/week), supplement use, and relationship status to help us to describe the individuals surveyed across the research.
- *Intervention/exposure*: We noted the type of drive for muscularity questionnaire participants had completed along with measures of reliability.
- *Context*: We determined whether participants were students or non-students.
- *Outcomes*: We recorded the

correlations between the drive for muscularity and anaerobic exercise, aerobic exercise, disordered eating, exercise dependence, supplement use, and McCreary and Sasse's (2000) Drive for Muscularity behaviour subscale.

Using the extraction sheet

We set up the code sheet in Excel to let us keep the information in one place, allow ease of communication between the two people undertaking extraction, and to avoid the double handling of information involved in paper-based systems. The spreadsheet allowed each primary investigation and independent sample within the studies to have at least one row. Some studies, for example, had more than one independent sample and participants were sometimes segregated according to gender, sexual orientation, or education level and their data were analysed separately. Further, some independent samples had more than one row because they had completed more than one drive for muscularity measure. Prior to data extraction, we determined rules to ensure the independence of the analysed effect sizes (e.g., only one effect size from each independent sample was included in an analysis).

Columns in the spreadsheet were labelled according to the information they contained and grouped to keep related information together. For example, the initial columns contained study and independent sample identifiers, such as the first author's name, year of study, and sample code to help with data management. Additional information included citation details, results from backward and forward searches, the inclusion/exclusion decision, and reasons for exclusion. The additional information was recorded to help us construct a PRISMA flowchart, keep all the information in one file, and easily add studies that were published after completing the search. Although the spreadsheet was adequate for the project, given the number of drive for muscularity studies now available, we would move to using dedicated review software if we were to update the review.

The recording of effect size is another area where we could improve our data extraction. We only recorded the effect size on the spreadsheet. Sometimes, however, we had to estimate or compute an effect size, because it was not presented in the original report. If we were to update the review, we would include columns where we would record detail about how we estimated effect sizes to avoid having to go back to the original source.

Two copies of the spreadsheet were created because two reviewers extracted data independently and differences were resolved through discussion and reference to source material. We calculated the percentage agreement at 94% and most of the differences that emerged arose because of ambiguity in the original source, such as variation in the reporting of sample size or internal reliability. In cases where we could not make an informed decision, we consulted the original authors and if we received no response we removed the study from the analysis. We also had to contact authors because a number of the original reports did not contain the information we needed. Not all researchers were able to supply the requested information and a number of studies that were relevant to the review were excluded for lack of detail.

Final reflections

We used Field and Gillett's (2010) syntax to analyse the data in both SPSS and R. The Excel spreadsheet allowed for the seamless transfer of the information from the data extraction spreadsheet to SPSS and R. If we update the review, using systematic review software would eliminate the need to transfer data across different packages. The Excel spreadsheet was useful, however, because it allowed us to easily format the evidence table and make our work transparent.

Summary

Extraction can be time-consuming and some investigators suggest the task could be automated through the use of technology based around natural language processing techniques (Jonnalagadda, Goyal, & Huffman, 2015). Existing systems, however, are not of sufficient quality to replace or even complement adequately human involvement (Jonnalagadda et al., 2015; Tsafnat et al., 2014). Until the day that Skynet pushes the button, people will bear the brunt of the effort in data extraction. The focus of this chapter has been on helping investigators develop transparent, methodical procedures to minimize the effort to secure the information on which the findings of their reviews will be based. Before exploring ways to analyse and synthesize the extracted data (▶ Chapter 9), the next chapter discusses ways to critically appraise the research from which the information was collected.

7

❓ Learning Exercises

1. Locate two systematic reviews in your discipline and read their methods and results section. From the information contained try to recreate their data extraction code sheet. Based on your re-creation:

   a. Can you arrange the items to reflect the data extraction purposes discussed in this chapter?

   b. Which information seems to be collected to answer the review question directly and which items contributed to providing contextual information?

   c. Do you think the authors could have collected additional information to help answer their question or provide contextual details?

   d. Could information have been extracted in an alternative format? (Regarding quantitative data, for example, if some items involved dichotomous responses, might continuous or ordinal information have been more useful? If themes were recorded from qualitative research, would direct quotes have been desirable?)

2. Based on the information contained in the proposal you developed in ▶ Chapter 2:

   a. Develop a data extraction code sheet and code book.

   b. Ask a relevant colleague or mentor to provide feedback.

   c. Pilot test the code sheet on a small number of papers likely to be part of your final sample of evidence.

   d. Based on the data extracted, develop results that might mirror the findings as you anticipate they will appear in your review.

   e. Evaluate the adequacy of the code sheet. (For example, are changes needed so you obtain the information needed to answer your review question?)

References

Booth, A., Sutton, A., & Papaioannou, D. (2016). *Systematic approaches to a successful literature review* (2nd ed.). Thousand Oaks, CA: Sage.

Borenstein, M., Hedges, L. V., Higgins, J. P. T., & Rothstein, H. R. (2009). *Introduction to meta-analysis.* Chichester, UK: Wiley.

Brown, S. A., Upchurch, S. L., & Acton, G. J. (2003). A framework for developing a coding scheme for meta-analysis. *Western Journal of Nursing Research, 25,* 205–222. ▶ https://doi.org/10.1177/0193945902250038.

Brunton, J., Graziosi, S., & Thomas, J. (2017). Tools and technologies for information management. In D. Gough, S. Oliver, & J. Thomas (Eds.), *An introduction to systematic reviews* (2nd ed., pp. 145–180). Thousand Oaks, CA: Sage.

Buscemi, N., Hartling, L., Vandermeer, B., Tjosvold, L., & Klassen, T. P. (2006). Single data extraction generated more errors than double data extraction in systematic reviews. *Journal of Clinical Epidemiology, 59,* 697–703. ▶ https://doi.org/10.1016/j.jclinepi.2005.11.010.

Chalmers, I., & Altman, D. G. (1995). *Systematic reviews.* London, UK: BMJ Publishing.

Craig, J. V., Bunn, D. K., Hayhoe, R. P., Appleyard, W. O., Lenaghan, E. A., & Welch, A. A. (2017). Relationship between the Mediterranean dietary pattern and musculoskeletal health in children, adolescents, and adults: Systematic review and evidence map. *Nutrition Reviews, 75,* 830–857. ▶ https://doi.org/10.1093/nutrit/nux042.

Elamin, M. B., Flynn, D. N., Bassler, D., Briel, M., Alonso-Coello, P., Karanicolas, P. J., … Montoria, V. M. (2009). Choice of data extraction tools for systematic reviews depends on resources and review complexity. *Journal of Clinical Epidemiology, 62,* 506–510. ▶ https://doi.org/10.1016/j.jclinepi.2008.10.016.

Field, A. P., & Gillett, R. (2010). How to do a meta-analysis. *British Journal of Mathematical and Statistical Psychology, 63,* 665–694. ▶ https://doi.org/10.1348/000711010X502733.

Gough, D., Oliver, S., & Thomas, J. (2017). Introducing systematic reviews. In D. Gough, S. Oliver, & J. Thomas (Eds.), *An introduction to systematic reviews* (2nd ed., pp. 1–17). Thousand Oaks, CA: Sage.

Gough, D., & Thomas, J. (2017). Commonality and diversity in reviews. In D. Gough, S. Oliver, & J. Thomas (Eds.), *An introduction to systematic reviews* (2nd ed., pp. 43–70). Thousand Oakes, CA: Sage.

Greenhalgh, T., Robert, G., Macfarlane, F., Bate, P., Kyriakidou, O., & Peacock, R. (2005). Storylines of research in diffusion of innovation: A meta-narrative approach to systematic review. *Social Science and Medicine, 61,* 417–430. ▶ https://doi.org/10.1016/j.socscimed.2004.12.001.

Higgins, J. P. T., & Deeks, J. J. (2011). Selecting studies and collecting data. In J. P. T. Higgins & S. Green (Eds.), *Cochrane handbook for systematic reviews of interventions.* The Cochrane Collaboration. Retrieved from ▶ www.cochrane-handbook.org.

Horton, J., Vandermeer, B., Hartling, L., Tjosvold, L., Klassen, T. P., & Buscemi, N. (2010). Systematic review data extraction: Cross-sectional study showed that experience did not increase accuracy. *Journal of Clinical Epidemiology, 63,* 289–298. ▶ https://doi.org/10.1016/j.jclinepi.2009.04.007.

Jonnalagadda, S. R., Goyal, P., & Huffman, M. D. (2015). Automating data extraction in systematic reviews: A systematic review. *Systematic Reviews, 4,* article 78. ▶ https://doi.org/10.1186/s13643-015-0066-7.

Langer, L. (2015). Sport for development—A systematic map of evidence from Africa. *South African Review of Sociology, 46,* 66–86. ▶ https://doi.org/10.1080/21528586.2014.989665.

Mathes, T., Klaßen, P., & Pieper, D. (2017). Frequency of data extraction errors and methods to increase data extraction quality: A methodological review. *BMC Medical Research Methodology, 17,* article 152. ▶ https://doi.org/10.1186/s12874-017-0431-4.

McCreary, D. R., & Sasse, D. K. (2000). An exploration of the drive for muscularity in adolescent boys and girls. *Journal of American College Health, 48,* 297–304. ▶ https://doi.org/10.1080/07448480009596271.

Miake-Lye, I. M., Hempel, S., Shanman, R., & Shekelle, P. G. (2016). What is an evidence map? A systematic review of published evidence maps and their definitions, methods, and products. *Systematic Reviews, 5*, article 28. ► https://doi.org/10.1186/s13643-016-0204-x.

Munoz, S. R., & Bangdiwala, S. I. (1997). Interpretation of Kappa and B statistics measures of agreement. *Journal of Applied Statistics, 24,* 105–112. ► https://doi.org/10.1080/02664769723918.

Parkhill, A. F., Clavisi, O., Pattuwage, L., Chau, M., Turner, T., Bragge, P., & Gruen, R. (2011). Searches for evidence mapping: Effective, shorter, cheaper. *Journal of the Medical Library Association, 99*, 157–160. ► https://doi.org/10.3163/1536-5050.99.2.008.

Paterson, B. L., Thorne, S. E., Canam, C., & Jillings, C. (2001). *Meta-study of qualitative health research: A practical guide to meta-analysis and meta-synthesis.* Thousand Oaks, CA: Sage.

Petticrew, M., & Roberts, H. (2006). *Systematic reviews in the social sciences: A practical guide.* Malden, MA: Blackwell.

Salmond, S., & Cooper, A. C. (2017). Steps in the systematic review process. In C. Holly, S. Salmond, & M. Saimbert (Eds.), *Comprehensive systematic review for advanced practice nursing* (2nd ed., pp. 17–38). New York, NY: Springer.

Shokraneh, F., & Adams, C. E. (2017). Increasing value and reducing waste in data extraction for systematic reviews: Tracking data in data extraction forms. *Systematic Reviews, 6*, article 153. ► https://doi.org/10.1186/s13643-017-0546-z.

Sutcliffe, K., Oliver, S., & Richardson, M. (2017). Describing and analysing studies. In D. Gough, S. Oliver, & J. Thomas (Eds.), *An introduction to systematic reviews* (2nd ed., pp. 123–144). Thousand Oaks, CA: Sage.

Tod, D., & Edwards, C. (2015). A meta-analysis of the drive for muscularity's relationships with exercise behaviour, disordered eating, supplement consumption, and exercise dependence. *International Review of Sport and Exercise Psychology, 8,* 185–203. ► https://doi.org/10.1080/1750984X.2015.1052089.

Tsafnat, G., Glasziou, P., Choong, M. K., Dunn, A., Galgani, F., & Coiera, E. (2014). Systematic review automation technologies. *Systematic Reviews, 3*, article 74. ► https://doi.org/10.1186/2046-4053-3-74.

7

Critical Appraisal

Learning Objectives

After reading this chapter, you should be able to:
- Define critical appraisal.
- Distinguish between bias and quality.
- Detail the reasons for critical appraisal.
- Describe the major types of research in your discipline.
- Critically appraise a body of research.
- Select criteria for appraising qualitative research.

Introduction

I have been fortunate to have helped charities and other organizations evaluate their public exercise interventions. Sometimes, these bodies have approached me and my colleagues after they have almost completed running the intervention and have realized they need to assess if it has been effective. These organizations view evaluation as something that is completed at the end of a project. The quality of an evaluation, however, is normally higher if people start planning and collecting information before the beginning of an intervention. For example, to decide if an exercise programme enhances people's mental well-being, it is helpful to know how good they felt about themselves before starting.

Similarly, some people think critically appraising research is a discrete step in a systematic review, conducted after the search, before the analysis, and possibly alongside data extraction. Although the formal in-depth assessment of individual studies may occur after the search and before analysis, reviewers benefit from planning and undertaking critical appraisal earlier in the journey. For example, formulating the inclusion and exclusion criteria encourages individuals to consider the external validity of relevant primary research. External validity refers to the degree that a study is relevant for the population of interest in a review (Booth, Sutton, & Papaioannou, 2016). Investigators might also consider the types of research designs suitable to the project and tailor their inclusion and exclusion criteria to reflect their judgements, such as focusing on randomized controlled trials for reviews on intervention effectiveness. As a second example, researchers may critically appraise seminal or notable studies when developing a review protocol to help them identify suitable critical appraisal criteria for the formal assessment of located research. As with the evaluation of exercise programmes, considering critical appraisal at the beginning of the project likely leads to more fruitful results than if left till the end. In the current chapter, I define critical appraisal; differentiate quality from bias; explain why appraisal is undertaken; overview major types of research in sport, exercise, and physical activity; present steps for conducting appraisal; and address qualitative research evaluation.

What Is Critical Appraisal?

Critical appraisal is "the process of carefully and systematically examining research to judge its trustworthiness, and its value and relevance in a particular context" (Burls, 2009, p. 1). Evaluating the rigour, merit, and applicability of research underpins sound evidence-based practice (Amonette, English, & Kraemer, 2016). Sport, exercise, and physical activity practitioners typically wish to provide high-quality services to individuals, groups, and communities. Science has a role in determining which interventions and ways of working with people are effective, safe, ethical, and humane. Research, however, varies in quality, type, and applicability. Critical appraisal allows sport, exercise, and physical activity scientists and practitioners to determine the level of confidence they can have in a body of work to guide decision-making. Without a critical attitude and commitment to relying on the best evidence available, professionals in our field may provide ineffective interventions that do not help, and may even harm, recipients of those services (Chalmers & Altman, 1995).

Further, critical appraisal and relying on scientific evidence are core values that set sport, exercise, and physical activity professionals apart from other service providers. One feature of a profession is having access to a specialist body of literature and tools (Winter & Collins, 2016). Without a sound base of scientific knowledge to guide practice, our discipline fails to be a profession, and practitioners are no different from a host of other self-proclaimed experts, snake oil salesmen, and charlatans vying for people's attention, public funding, and private or corporate disposal income. To rely on scientific knowledge we need to understand what research is credible. Critical appraisal allows professionals to (a) decide if scientific research is trustworthy, (b) make sense of the results, and (c) understand what those findings mean for the situations in which they work (Amonette et al., 2016; Burls, 2009).

There are three components to critical appraisal, and they involve reviewers assessing a primary study's methodological rigour, suitability, and relevance (Liabo, Gough, & Harden, 2017). First, rigour refers to method soundness or internal validity. Numerous tools exist to help assess rigour, and reviewers can select ones suited to the designs of the studies they are examining. For example, the Cochrane Risk of Bias tool is tailored towards randomized controlled trials (Higgins, Altman, & Sterne, 2017). Tools for different designs are available from the internet, such as from the Critical Appraisal Skills Programme's website (▶ https://casp-uk.net/casp-tools-checklists/) or the Joanna Briggs Institute (▶ http://joannabriggs.org/).

Second, design suitability deals with the match between a study's method and the review question (Liabo et al., 2017). Experimental, but not observational research, for example, would be suitable for reviews on intervention effectiveness. Decisions about method suitability are often made during the search and are reflected in the inclusion and exclusion criteria.

Third, study relevance considers how well the investigation contributes to the review question and context (Liabo et al., 2017). Sometimes relevance is addressed at stages other than the critical appraisal step, such as during the search when the inclusion and exclusion criteria help screen out unsuitable studies. If undertaken during the formal critical appraisal step, the assessment of relevance is influenced by the review's purpose and context. For example, if a review is designed to underpin practice guidelines for using psychological interventions with athletes, investigators would consider the primary study's participants (e.g., level of athlete) and context (e.g., were the dependent variable data collected during or away from competition?). Knowing that most researchers have examined novices, and have assessed dependent variables in controlled environments, helps reviewers in framing the boundaries of their recommendations.

What Is the Difference Between Quality and Bias?

When considering critical appraisal it is helpful to distinguish between quality and bias. In some sport, exercise, and physical activity reviews, quality is equated to bias although they are different (Petticrew & Roberts, 2006). To illustrate, the Cochrane Collaboration defines bias as "systematic error, or deviation from the truth, in results or inferences" (Higgins et al., 2017, p. 8.3), whereas quality refers to "the extent to which study authors conducted their research to the highest possible standards" (Higgins et al., 2017, p. 8.4). The Cochrane Collaboration separates bias from quality for several reasons:

- Primary research may be undertaken to the highest standards possible, but still contain bias. For example, in randomized controlled trials of self-talk on sports performance, blinding participants is not generally meaningful. Most participants are likely to realize the purpose of the study once they have been asked to utter different types of self-statements from pre- to post-test, and their insight may influence their performance. Although bias is present, the researchers may still have done the best that was possible given the topic being examined.
- In sport, exercise, and physical activity research, some indicators of quality are unlikely to directly introduce bias, such as obtaining ethical approval, consulting stakeholders, or adhering to reporting standards.
- Focusing on bias helps address the tension between a study's reporting and implementation quality, although reviewers are still reliant on reports to evaluate the investigations.

Bias can be assessed by considering a study's internal validity, whereas quality is a broader and more subjective idea (Petticrew & Roberts, 2006). Although quality includes bias, it also embraces other yardsticks that the intended audience may consider relevant. In social care contexts, for example, relevant quality criteria may include (Pawson, Boaz, Grayson, Long, & Barnes, 2003):

- *Transparency*: Is the study clear on how the knowledge was produced?
- *Accuracy*: Does the study rely on relevant evidence to generate the knowledge?
- *Purpose*: Did the study employ suitable methods?
- *Utility*: Does the study answer the questions?
- *Propriety*: Is the study legal and ethical?
- *Accessibility*: Can intended audiences understand the study?
- *Specificity*: Does the study conform to the standards for the type of knowledge generated?

Pawson et al.'s criteria show that a study's quality is influenced by more than its inherent features, but also by the context in which it resides and the target audience.

Why Undertake Critical Appraisal?

Perfect high-quality studies that are free from bias do not exist. Primary studies vary in quality for a host of reasons. The influence of bias, for example, (a) ranges from trivial to substantial, (b) leads to both under and overestimation of effects, and (c) cannot always be identified by researchers (Higgins et al., 2017). Critical appraisal is not a search for the perfect study, but an evaluation of what the available evidence allows us to have confidence in and believe (Booth et al., 2016; Liabo et al., 2017). The results from a critical appraisal may also inform a sensitivity analysis, or the evaluation of how a review's findings change as studies with particular design features or biases are included or excluded (Petticrew & Roberts, 2006).

Critical appraisal helps to ensure transparency and consistency in the assessment of primary research. Further, people who use critical appraisal tools, compared with those who do not, are more consistent in their ratings, apply more suitable criteria, and are less influenced by personal biases and subject-specific knowledge (Crowe, Sheppard, & Campbell, 2011; MacAuley, McCrum, & Brown, 1998). People, including researchers, are often not reliable or self-aware decision makers, and they fall prey to numerous cognitive biases (Kahneman, 2012). Example cognitive biases that appear in research include (Nuzzo, 2015):

- Collecting evidence to support a favoured hypothesis, not searching for opposing information, and ignoring rival explanations (*hypothesis myopia*).
- Identifying random patterns in the evidence and treating them as meaningful (*the Texas sharpshooter*).
- Checking unexpected results but not anticipated findings (*asymmetric attention*).
- Suggesting explanations after analysing results to rationalize what has been found (*just-so storytelling*).

Ways to counter biases in systematic reviewing include (a) considering and testing rival hypotheses, (b) registering protocols to declare data extraction and analysis plans publically before undertaking reviews, (c) collaborating with individuals with opposing beliefs, (d) having multiple people undertake various steps independently of each other and comparing results, and (e) asking stakeholders and disinterested individuals to offer feedback on the final report before making it publically available.

Inconsistent critical appraisal can lead to one or both of two results:

» At one extreme of the spectrum, where data are accepted on face value (no appraisal), the risk of a type I error (accepting evidence of efficacy when the intervention does not work or causes harm) is high, and that of a type II error (discarding evidence when the intervention actually works) is low. At the other extreme (excessive scrutiny) the risk of a type II error is great. (Woolf, 2000, p. 1082)

Being overly critical or unduly accepting may lead to inaccurate results or interpretations of primary research. The flow on effects may be poor practice recommendations and harm to people involved in sport, exercise, and physical activity. Competent reviewers are not attempting to criticize primary research to rationalize exclusion or find fault, but instead they are attempting to ascertain omissions, errors, and biases "that are large enough to affect how the result of the study should be interpreted" (Petticrew & Roberts, 2006, p. 128). To engage in critical appraisal well, it is helpful for reviewers to be familiar with the types of research that occur within their domains of interest.

Major Types of Research in Sport, Exercise, and Physical Activity

To help complete high quality reviews of primary research, it is useful to be aware of the types of studies that get conducted in an investigator's domain (Boland, Cherry, & Dickson, 2017; Booth et al., 2016). ◻ Table 8.1 presents some common research designs in sport, exercise, and physical activity literature. Our field, however, consists of several sub-disciplines from the physical and biological domains to the social sciences and humanities. Studies vary a great deal across the sub-disciplines and investigators from these areas use different labels to identify similar types of research. Despite the discrepancies, there are consistent ways by which research can be described. Understanding these variations helps identify the strengths and weaknesses of the existing research designs and can inform critical appraisal. Briefly, some of these features include:

◻ **Table 8.1**   Common types of research in sport, exercise, and physical activity

Type of research	Example question
Experiment A study in which investigators manipulate the independent variable to assess its influence on a dependent variable, while ideally controlling other variables	What is the influence of a particular type of training programme, compared with no intervention, on swing mechanics in golf?
Cross-sectional survey Investigators collect data from a sample of individuals at a single time point to describe some phenomena	What are the body shape and composition profiles of New Zealand high school female netball players?
Longitudinal survey Researchers collect data from a sample of individuals at multiple time points to assess how variables change over time	How does physical activity participation change as children proceed through various grades at school?
Case control studies Investigators compare individuals with or without particular characteristics on a range of variables	How do people with depression vary in their exercise and nutrition habits compared with individuals without depression?
Case study The in-depth examination of a single person, group, organization, or event that typically involves the collection of various types of data to provide a holistic description	What is the culture of the St Louis Arch Rival Roller Derby league?

- *Experimental versus descriptive research*: Experimental studies involve scientists intervening in people's lives, as illustrated in randomized controlled trials. During descriptive research, investigators do not intervene but attempt to observe and document what is occurring with as little intrusion as possible, such as when they undertake prospective cohort studies. Experimental studies allow investigators to explore causal relationships, but often do so under artificial conditions. Descriptive research is less capable of examining causality, but may be able to collect data in real-world situations.

- *Control versus uncontrolled*: A controlled study involves attempts to rule out rival hypotheses. In an experiment, for example, random allocation helps to ensure that participants in separate conditions are equivalent regarding their personal characteristics. In descriptive research, investigators may also attempt to control confounding variables, using strategies such as case-control designs, strict participant inclusion criteria, or statistical techniques to assess covariance.

- *Cross-sectional versus longitudinal studies*: Cross-sectional studies involve collecting data on one occasion, such as in one-shot surveys of attitudes. In longitudinal studies repeated measures of the same variables are undertaken at different time points. A pre- and post-test experiment is a longitudinal study, although the intervening time between measurements can vary from seconds to years. Cross-sectional studies are often easier and cheaper to undertake, whereas longitudinal studies allow a stronger basis for prediction and for hypothesizing possible causal relationships (that need to be tested in experiments).

- *Prospective versus retrospective studies*: Prospective studies are forward focused. Participants are identified and followed over time with variables being measured after people agreed to participate. Retrospective studies are backward focused, with attempts to assess what was happening before people agreed to participate. Recall bias can be a limitation with retrospective studies, although they can be easier and cheaper to undertake than prospective studies.

- *Within versus between group designs*: Comparison between people can be undertaken when there are multiple groups, such as comparing intervention with contrast conditions in experimental studies (between group design). Comparisons between conditions can be made using one group if participants have experienced the various interventions, ideally in a random or counterbalanced order (within group design).

- *Random versus non-random allocation*: The advantage of using random allocation in a between group design is that differences among participants can be distributed equally given a sufficient sample size. With non-random allocation, differences among participants may result in confounding factors that influence findings. When participants serve as their own control in a within group design, the order they are exposed to the conditions may influence results. Random allocation of conditions, or the more common strategy of counterbalancing, avoids order effects.

- *Random versus non-random selection*: During random selection, individuals from an identified population have an equal chance of being invited into the study. Given a sufficient sample size, the participants in the study will be representative of the population. Random selection allows researchers to generalize findings back to the population. Non-random selection may result in samples that do not represent the population.

— **Blind versus open studies**: In blind studies, participants are unaware of the condition or exposure they have received, whereas they will know or be able to guess in an open study. In double-blind studies, both the participants and the researchers with whom they interact are unaware of the condition or exposure. Although blind studies reduce participant or researcher effects from influencing the study, they are sometimes not possible or ethical in many sport, exercise, and physical activity topic areas.

The ways above in which research varies are not mutually exclusive. For example, experimental studies can (a) involve either random or non-random allocation, (b) adopt a between or within group design, (c) vary in whether a control group or condition is included, and (d) be cross-sectional or longitudinal. Although the list is brief and not exhaustive it does introduce the common ways along which studies differ from each other across the sport, exercise, and physical activity subdomains. Awareness of these differences can help reviewers become familiar with the typical strengths and weaknesses associated with research in their topics of interest. Understanding the common research types helps reviewers determine what studies are relevant to their reviews, select suitable inclusion and exclusion criteria, and identify useful data extraction and critical appraisal instruments.

Undertaking Critical Appraisal of a Body of Research

Critical appraisal can be divided into a number of steps to help reviewers undertake the task in a rigorous systematic fashion (Goldstein, Venker, & Weng, 2017), including Aim, Attributes, Acquisition, Arrangement or Administration, and Application.

Aim   Begin by detailing the aim or purpose of critical appraisal and visualizing what information is needed to achieve the objective. For example, is the assessment of bias or internal validity sufficient for the project, or is there a need to evaluate other quality-related benchmarks, such as adherence to reporting standards? To determine the aim of the appraisal, it is useful to consider the intended audiences and what criteria they are likely to find credible and relevant. Also, survey the types of evidence that will be evaluated. Generally, using an appraisal tool that is suitable for the type of primary study being assessed is preferable to employing a generic instrument (Boland et al., 2017). The information from a specific tool will be more useful for interpreting the review's findings than data from a general checklist.

Attributes   Attributes refer to the logistics of critical appraisal, for example, when, what, who, where, and how is it going to happen. For example, when will appraisal take place? Will it be done concurrently with data extraction or can some aspects occur at other times? Regarding the people who will undertake critical appraisal, it is useful to consider their level of training and discipline-specific expertise. For example, it may be useful to include people who are experts in research methodology, the content area of the project, or both.

Reviewers also benefit from considering their selection of critical appraisal tools carefully. Many tools exist, but their content often does not overlap and they can lead to different evaluations of quality (Armijo-Olivo, Stiles, Hagen, Biondo, & Cummings,

2012). Additionally, most tools are untested and lack clear guidelines for their use (Katrak, Bialocerkowski, Massy-Westropp, Kumar, & Grimmer, 2004; Sanderson, Tatt, & Higgins, 2007). Furthermore, many tools focus almost exclusively on methodological rigour and authors may overlook that critical appraisal also includes a study's relevance and suitability for the review (Liabo et al., 2017).

Acquisition Acquisition refers to the business of extracting the information from individual studies, using the selected tools or checklists. One key point during acquisition is ensuring consistency across reviewers or within an individual over time. Decision shift or wobble, for example, occurs when reviewers' application of the checklist varies as they proceed through the primary research, such as becoming less tolerant or more flexible as they near the end of the activity. Shift and wobble may occur if the items on the checklist are vague or reviewers do not understand them. Similar to data extraction, strategies to encourage consistency include (a) having multiple people complete acquisition independently and then compare results, (b) having team meetings to help individuals gain a shared understanding of how to apply criteria, and (c) subjecting results to an audit trail by a disinterested individual to identify areas of inconsistency. To demonstrate the absence of decision wobble, teams can present reliability statistics.

Arrangement or administration Critical appraisal can generate a large amount of information. A systematic way of organizing and presenting the information allows reviewers to make sense of the results and use it to inform their evaluation of the research. Cochrane reviews, for example, contain a table that details how investigators rated each primary study against each risk of bias item. A traffic light system is used where green represents adherence, amber a lack of clarity, and red nonadherence. The table is typically supplemented with a graph which presents the percentage of studies with each rating level for each risk of bias item. The table and graph help readers assess the quality of the body of literature and use the information to help interpret the review findings. Cochrane reviews are open access, so you can search their library to view examples.

Application Often reviewers do not use their critical appraisal results to inform their interpretation of the research or present them in ways helpful to readers (Katikireddi, Egan, & Petticrew, 2015). Although some people report the information without discussion, a better practice is to use the information to help interpret the review's findings. For example, if a review finds that five studies suggest an intervention is effective, readers are likely to think it is promising. If reviewers add that the five studies were of poor quality, readers will change their opinions. Alternatively if the five studies were of good quality, readers' confidence in the intervention will increase.

Some authors may use the results to exclude studies deemed to be of poor quality (Southward, Rutherfurd-Markwick, & Ali, 2018), although doing so prevents the community from examining how quality influences the results or identifying typical limitations that need to be resolved (Card, 2012). A better practice in some situations is to undertake a sensitivity analysis where reviewers examine how quality markers are related to the results (Higgins et al., 2017).

Suitable Criteria for Appraising Qualitative Research

Researchers in sport, exercise, and physical activity have debated how to critically appraise qualitative research since its introduction to the field. Equally, the topic of how to evaluate qualitative work has generated similar discussions among systematic reviewers in health care and related disciplines. Opinions range from (a) the belief that it is acceptable to use traditional scientific quality criteria to (b) the argument that critical appraisal is not possible because of the reliance on subjectivity (Petticrew & Roberts, 2006). Appraising primary research is a core value in systematic reviewing, and assessing qualitative research is possible (and necessary) to allow us to gauge the level of confidence we can have in the knowledge that authors generate (Carroll & Booth, 2015; Patton, 2015). An adequate appraisal of qualitative investigations, or any type of research, however, occurs if suitable criteria are applied. Quantitative yardsticks, such as validity and reliability, are not apt criteria to guide evaluation of qualitative investigations (Salmond & Porter, 2017).

Identifying suitable criteria by which to assess qualitative studies has occupied the attention of systematic reviewers in recent years, as the ways to synthesize evidence has broadened and diversified. Authors have generated various checklists, assessment tools, and lists of questions in their efforts to standardize procedures, reflecting their attempts to ensure transparency and rigour when reviewing literature (Carroll & Booth, 2015). Although laudable, there are shortcomings to the theory underlying some of these tools.

Systematic reviewers often attempt to develop criteria that can be applied to all qualitative research. When writing about how to critically appraise qualitative research, systematic review authors normally go as far as highlighting the epistemological, ontological, methodological, axiological, and rhetorical differences between qualitative and quantitative investigations (Yilmaz, 2013, provides a clear discussion). Such presentations, however, typically fail to differentiate among the various qualitative traditions and treat them as essentially the same method. The various qualitative methods (e.g., grounded theory, narrative analysis, ethnography), however, have different central questions, purposes, assumptions, procedures, and outputs (Patton, 2015). Just as it is unsuitable to apply quantitative criteria to qualitative work, it can be as equally nonsensical to use one set of benchmarks for all the different flavours of naturalistic inquiry. Instead, reviewers who tailor their criteria to match the type of study they are critiquing are likely to gain a better understanding of the work than if they adopt a universal set of benchmarks. As an illustration, Patton (2015) discusses the quality standards associated with several viewpoints that underpin qualitative research:

- **The traditional positivistic viewpoint.** Qualitative research informed by a traditional positivistic viewpoint contains words and phrases such as hypothesis testing, variables, validity, and generalizability. The aim of these qualitative studies is to detail phenomenon accurately so that descriptions correspond closely to reality. These investigators emphasize rigour, technical expertise, and systematic procedures for data collection and analysis. To reflect their point of view, they draw on traditional science criteria including validity and reliability, as exemplified through attempts to measure intercoder reliability or kappa coefficients.

- *The social constructivist viewpoint.* Investigators informed by a social constructionist mindset assume that people create their social worlds. These researchers embrace subjectivity as integral to understanding human affairs. The aim is to offer alternative understandings of social phenomena and stimulate dialogue rather than propose singular truths. Examples of criteria associated with social knowledge construction include authenticity, triangulation, reflexivity, praxis, and rich description.
- *The artistic or evocative viewpoint.* When undertaking artistic qualitative research, investigators try to engage with, connect to, move, provoke, or stimulate the audience. Artistic qualitative researchers strive to show the emotional and behavioural dimensions to their findings, as well as cognitive components. Example artistic criteria include aesthetics, creativity, expression, connection, and stimulation.
- *The critical change viewpoint.* Those people conducting qualitative research informed by a critical change standpoint try to go beyond just studying a phenomenon to questioning the associated human consequences, with a view to stimulating political and social change. Critical theorists use their work to critique society, challenge those in authority, raise awareness, and adjust power imbalances for the benefit of the less fortunate. Criteria by which individuals evaluate their work include consequential validity, praxis, raising awareness of injustices, and identifying inequality and discrimination.

Conversations between quantitative and qualitative researchers can be laden with misunderstanding and frustration if they fail to acknowledge that they advocate different assumptions, purposes, and values. For example, individuals operating from a quantitative view may value knowledge advancement and do not think they have a responsibility to instigate change. Critical change-minded folks, however, may deemphasize theory development but value real-world impact. The same frustrations and misunderstandings can emerge during conversations between individuals operating from different qualitative schools because they also vary in their values and beliefs.

Systematic reviewers may find that many of the available checklists to guide appraisal of qualitative research do not allow a fair and reasonable evaluation of the primary studies they locate. Instead, tailoring their checklists to reflect the underlying methodology of the primary research yields a meaningful end result. In addition, quality and credibility intersect with audiences and the project's intended purposes (Patton, 2015). A qualitative study's credibility is not an inherent permanent attribute, but instead is a dynamic characteristic that varies across audiences and time (Burke, 2016).

Two questions can help guide reviewers when critically appraising qualitative research. First, is this a good study in light of its grounding tradition (ethnography, grounded theory, narrative analysis)? Second, in what ways does this study provide findings that can contribute to the current review? To answer the first question, reviewers need to tailor their criteria to match those of the primary study's underlying methodological stance (e.g., traditional science, social construction, etc.).

The answer to the second question involves considering the match between the review purpose and theoretical orientation of the primary research. The different theoretical traditions in qualitative research have different foci and aims (Patton, 2015). For example, the central focus of ethnographic research is describing the culture of a group of people.

The central question in positivistic work is what is really going on in the real world? In phenomenology, the guiding aim is to describe the meaning, structure, and essence of people's experience with a phenomenon. In narrative research, investigators ask: what does this narrative reveal about the person and world from which it was constructed?

Primary qualitative research will likely contribute optimally to a review when it matches the project's theoretical orientation. For example, if the review question emphasizes understanding a group's culture then ethnographic primary research will likely contribute more than grounded theory research. The previous sentence does not imply that grounded theory studies cannot contribute to reviews about culture, only that on balance ethnographies are likely to be more helpful, because their major focus is the examination of a group's shared beliefs and behaviours. As an analogy, in meta-analyses reviewers often separate out experimental designs from descriptive designs. Descriptive research may give insights into the strength of a relationship, but provide weak evidence of causality.

The match, however, between a review and primary research is not always simple or straightforward. Review questions can be complex or broad enough that research from various traditions is needed to make meaningful contributions. Although reviewers of quantitative research may be able to develop inclusion and exclusion based around research design, the same may not always be suitable for qualitative research.

8

Chapter Case Example: Does Resistance Training Frequency Influence Muscular Strength Gains?

In 2018, Grgic, Schoenfeld, Davies, Lazinica, Krieger, and Pedisic, reported a systematic review and meta-analysis in which they examined the influence of resistance training frequency on muscular strength gains. If you would like to obtain a copy, it was published on pages 1207–1220 in *Sports Medicine*, Vol. 48, and similar to much research these days you may be able to obtain an author's copy from places such as Researchgate. In this chapter, I will focus on the way the authors addressed critical appraisal.

Study Purpose
The article's purpose was: "(1) to perform a systematic review of the studies that compare different RT [resistance training] frequencies while assessing muscular strength outcomes; (2) to quantify the findings with a meta-analysis; and (3) to draw evidence based conclusions guiding exercise program design" (Grgic et al., 2018, p. 1208). The purpose is not presented in the PICO format, but later on, in the method, the authors clarify that:

— *Participants* had to have been humans free of pre-existing chronic disease or injury.

— *Interventions* had to have been resistance training programmes using dynamic exercises lasting at least four weeks.

— Regarding *comparison*, there were no standard control conditions. Instead, the most common comparison involved comparing two with three training sessions per week.

— *Outcomes* included a 1 repetition maximum test, an isokinetic test, or an isometric test, with the bench press and leg press being the most common movements assessed.

Critical Appraisal Process
The authors used Downs and Black's (1998) checklist to assess the located studies. The checklist contains 27 items designed to assess features related to reporting, external

validity, internal validity, and statistical power. Grgic et al. (2018) added two additional items focused on resistance training adherence and supervision. For each item, studies were given one point for satisfying the criteria or no points for either not meeting the criteria or not providing sufficient details to allow the investigators to make a decision. Reviewers then calculated a total score, with possible marks ranging from 0 to 29. To assist interpretation, the authors rated studies as *good quality* if they scored 21–29, as *moderate quality* for scores of 11–20, and as *poor quality* for totals below 11. To undertake critical appraisal, two individuals rated each study independently of each other and then resolved differences through discussion.

Many reviews in sport, exercise, and physical activity focus only on assessing internal validity, despite it being only one aspect of critical appraisal. Grgic et al.'s (2018) examination of external validity, reporting, statistical power, and two features of intervention fidelity provides a broader assessment of the primary research. The calculation of a total score is a contested practice, however. Studies might achieve the same total score but for different reasons. Total scores do not allow readers to compare and contrast the studies in terms of the specific critical appraisal features. The total score may not be as helpful as knowing how studies rated on individual items. Such information is available, however, because Grgic et al. presented a table that detailed how studies rated on each item of the critical appraisal checklist.

Critical Appraisal Results

The average critical appraisal score was 18, and ranged from 13 to 22. Regarding cut-off scores, four studies were rated a good, the rest as moderate, and none as poor. The strongest feature of the critical appraisal process in the paper is the second table in the report in which the authors present how each study fared against the items on Downs and Black's (1998) checklist. The information reveals on which items all or the vast majority of primary studies performed well and the ones on which they could have improved. With respect to reporting standards, for example, all or the vast majority of studies clearly described the purpose statement, the main outcomes, the participants, interventions, and main findings. There was much greater variation in the reporting of confounding variables, adverse events, and exact probability values. Regarding internal validity, most studies did not describe, or provide sufficient information, regarding blinding, double blinding, and the analysis of confounding. The value of Grgic et al.'s (2018) second table in the report is that it deflects the readers' attention away from focusing on individual studies and encourages them to consider the body of work as a whole and explore trends across the primary investigations. The central focus of critical appraisal, as mentioned above, is to gauge how confident we can be in the review findings, based on the total evidence, rather than trying to identify outstanding studies, be they of extremely high or low quality.

The authors touched lightly on the critical appraisal to help them develop future research recommendations, including the tracking and reporting of adverse events, the presentation of adherence rates, and the supervision of resistance training programmes. It is largely left to the reader, however, to consider how the methodological strengths and weaknesses might have influenced results. It may have been insightful, for example, if the authors had undertaken a sensitivity analysis and explored how the results changed with the presence or absence of various quality markers, such as participant intervention compliance.

Summary

According to Stephen King (2000, p. 201), the novelist: "when you write a book, you spend day after day scanning and identifying the trees. When you're done, you have to step back and look at the forest." His words can be applied to critical appraisal in a systematic review. Evaluating research involves dissecting each study to a fine level of detail. All studies have limitations and critical appraisal will uncover their flaws. It is easy to become overly critical and believe no study is good enough, an attitude Sackett et al. (1997) labelled *critical appraisal nihilism*. Not all limitations, however, influence results and imperfect studies still contribute to our understanding of the world. The value of critical appraisal becomes clear when we step back from the granular details and examine the trends across a body of research. These trends allow us to make informed decisions about how much we can trust the findings from our review. The next chapter examines ways that we can synthesize primary research findings and make sense of the knowledge.

8

❷ Learning Exercises

1. Select a study on a topic that interests you. Visit the Critical Appraisal Skills Programme's (CASP; ▶ https://casp-uk.net/) and the Joanna Brigg's Institute's (▶ https://joannabriggs.org/) websites and obtain their critical appraisal tools relevant to the study that you decided to read. Read the study and then critically appraise it twice, once using the CASP tool and again with the Joanna Brigg's instrument. Compare the two tools:
   - Which seemed easier to use and had clearer instructions?
   - Did one helped you understand and evaluate the study more than the other?
   - Was there information missing from the tools that you thought needed to be added?
   - If asked for a recommendation, which tool would you suggest and why?

2. Having completed exercise 1, find another 4 studies on the same topic and appraise them using one of the above tools. Undertake the exercise with a friend.
   - Start by each of you appraising the studies independently of each other.
   - On completion, compare your findings and calculate how much you agreed on the results. Discuss and resolve variation and seek explanations for why you differed.
   - Together identify a way by which you could present the results in a visual manner that encapsulates the major trends, such as a table, chart, or figure.
   - To complete the exercise, use the results from the critical appraisal to judge how confident we can be in the five original studies' content findings.

3. Revisit the review protocol you have been developing. In light of the current chapter:
   - Identify and pilot a critical appraisal tool relevant to the evidence you will assess.
   - Make a decision about how you will handle the information and incorporate it into your project.
   - Update the protocol you wrote from ▶ Chapter 2.

References

Amonette, W. E., English, K. L., & Kraemer, W. J. (2016). *Evidence-based practice in exercise science: The six-step approach*. Champaign, IL: Human Kinetics.

Armijo-Olivo, S., Stiles, C. R., Hagen, N. A., Biondo, P. D., & Cummings, G. G. (2012). Assessment of study quality for systematic reviews: A comparison of the Cochrane collaboration risk of bias tool and the effective public health practice project quality assessment tool—Methodological research. *Journal of Evaluation in Clinical Practice, 18*, 12–18. ► https://doi.org/10.1111/j.1365-2753.2010.01516.X.

Boland, A., Cherry, G. M., & Dickson, R. (2017). *Doing a systematic review: A student's guide* (2nd ed.). Thousand Oaks, CA: Sage.

Booth, A., Sutton, A., & Papaioannou, D. (2016). *Systematic approaches to a successful literature review* (2nd ed.). Thousand Oaks, CA: Sage.

Burke, S. (2016). Rethinking 'validity' and 'trustworthiness' in qualitative inquiry: How might we judge the quality of qualitative research in sport and exercise sciences? In B. Smith & A. C. Sparkes (Eds.), *Routledge handbook of qualitative research in sport and exercise* (pp. 330–339). London, UK: Routledge.

Burls, A. (2009). *What is critical appraisal?* (2nd ed.). Newmarket, UK: Haywood Medical Communications.

Card, N. A. (2012). *Applied meta-analysis for social science research*. New York, NY: Guilford.

Carroll, C., & Booth, A. (2015). Quality assessment of qualitative evidence for systematic review and synthesis: Is it meaningful, and if so, how should it be performed? *Research Synthesis Methods, 6*, 149–154. ► https://doi.org/10.1002/jrsm.1128.

Chalmers, I., & Altman, D. G. (1995). *Systematic reviews*. London, UK: BMJ Publishing.

Crowe, M., Sheppard, L., & Campbell, A. (2011). Comparison of the effects of using the Crowe critical appraisal tool versus informal appraisal in assessing health research: A randomised trial. *International Journal of Evidence-Based Healthcare, 9*, 444–449. ► https://doi.org/10.1111/j.1744-1609.2011.00237.x.

Downs, S. H., & Black, N. (1998). The feasibility of creating a checklist for the assessment of the methodological quality both of randomised and non-randomised studies of health care interventions. *Journal of Epidemiology and Community Health, 52*, 377–384. ► https://doi.org/10.1136/jech.52.6.377.

Goldstein, A., Venker, E., & Weng, C. (2017). Evidence appraisal: A scoping review, conceptual framework, and research agenda. *Journal of the American Medical Informatics Association, 24*, 1192–1203. ► https://doi.org/10.1093/jamia/ocx050.

Grgic, J., Schoenfeld, B. J., Davies, T. B., Lazinica, B., Krieger, J. W., & Pedisic, Z. (2018). Effect of resistance training frequency on gains in muscular strength: A systematic review and meta-analysis. *Sports Medicine, 48*, 1207–1220. ► https://doi.org/10.1007/s40279-018-0872-x.

Higgins, J. P. T., Altman, D. G., & Sterne, J. A. C. (2017). Assessing risk of bias in included studies. In J. P. T. Higgins, R. Churchill, J. Chandler, & M. S. Cumpston (Eds.), *Cochrane handbook for systematic reviews of interventions* (version 5.2.0). Retrieved from ► www.training.cochrane.org/handbook.

Kahneman, D. (2012). *Thinking, fast and slow*. London, UK: Penguin.

Katikireddi, S. V., Egan, M., & Petticrew, M. (2015). How do systematic reviews incorporate risk of bias assessments into the synthesis of evidence? A methodological study. *Journal of Epidemiology and Community Health, 69*, 189–195. ► https://doi.org/10.1136/jech-2014-204711.

Katrak, P., Bialocerkowski, A. E., Massy-Westropp, N., Kumar, V. S. S., & Grimmer, K. A. (2004). A systematic review of the content of critical appraisal tools. *BMC Medical Research Methodology, 4*, article 22. ► https://doi.org/10.1186/1471-2288-4-22.

King, S. (2000). *On writing: A memoir of the craft*. New York, NY: Scribner.

Liabo, K., Gough, D., & Harden, A. (2017). Developing justifiable evidence claims. In D. Gough, S. Oliver, & J. Thomas (Eds.), *An introduction to systematic reviews* (2nd ed., pp. 251–277). Thousand Oaks, CA: Sage.

MacAuley, D., McCrum, E., & Brown, C. (1998). Randomised controlled trial of the READER method of critical appraisal in general practice. *British Medical Journal, 316*, 1134–1137. ► https://doi.org/10.1136/bmj.316.7138.1134.

Nuzzo, R. (2015). How scientists fool themselves—And how they can stop. *Nature News, 526*(7572), 182–185.

Patton, M. Q. (2015). *Qualitative research and evaluation methods* (4th ed.). Thousand Oaks, CA: Sage.

Pawson, R., Boaz, A., Grayson, L., Long, A., & Barnes, C. (2003). *Types and quality of knowledge in social care*. London, UK: Social Care Institute for Excellence.

Petticrew, M., & Roberts, H. (2006). *Systematic reviews in the social sciences: A practical guide*. Malden, MA: Blackwell.

Sackett, D. L., Richardson, S., Rosenberg, W., & Haynes, R. B. (1997). *Evidence-based medicine: How to practice and teach EBM*. Philadelphia, PA: WB Saunders Company.

Salmond, S., & Porter, S. (2017). Critical appraisal. In C. Holly, S. Salmond, & M. Saimbert (Eds.), *Comprehensive systematic review for advanced practice nursing* (2nd ed., pp. 173–189). New York, NY: Springer.

Sanderson, S., Tatt, I. D., & Higgins, J. P. T. (2007). Tools for assessing quality and susceptibility to bias in observational studies in epidemiology: A systematic review and annotated bibliography. *International Journal of Epidemiology, 36*, 666–676. ▶ https://doi.org/10.1093/ije/dym018.

Southward, K., Rutherford-Markwick, K. J., & Ali, A. (2018). The effect of acute caffeine ingestion on endurance performance: A systematic review and meta-analysis. *Sports Medicine, 48*, 1913–1928. ▶ https://doi.org/10.1007/s40279-018-0939-8.

Winter, S., & Collins, D. J. (2016). Applied sport psychology: A profession? *The Sport Psychologist, 30*, 89–96. ▶ https://doi.org/10.1123/tsp.2014-0132.

Woolf, S. H. (2000). Taking critical appraisal to extremes: The need for balance in the evaluation of evidence. *The Journal of Family Practice, 49*, 1081–1085.

Yilmaz, K. (2013). Comparison of quantitative and qualitative research traditions: Epistemological, theoretical, and methodological differences. *European Journal of Education, 48*, 311–325. ▶ https://doi.org/10.1111/ejed.12014.

8

Data Analysis and Synthesis

© The Author(s) 2019
D. Tod, *Conducting Systematic Reviews in Sport, Exercise, and Physical Activity*,
https://doi.org/10.1007/978-3-030-12263-8_9

Learning Objectives

After reading this chapter, you should be able to:
- Explain differences between data analysis and synthesis.
- Identify suitable analysis and synthesis methods for specific review purposes.
- Describe a generic framework to guide analysis and synthesis.
- Customize the generic framework to answer specific review questions.

Introduction

» Raw data is both an oxymoron and a bad idea; to the contrary, data should be cooked with care (Bowker, 2005, p. 183).

An exciting part of a systematic review is the analysis. Having obtained the literature and extracted the data, reviewers can now examine the information and answer their questions. There may be self-aggrandizing beliefs that you are making a contribution to human knowledge because you are moulding raw clay into a worthwhile or decorative object. As Bowker (2005) points out, however, the extracted information is not raw or uncooked. To prepare their studies for publication, researchers have had to make numerous decisions that have shaped and flavoured the information, just like farmers and grocers modify vegetables to increase their taste and attractiveness for consumers.

Understanding that data is not untainted, and that extraction, analysis, and interpretation are not neutral stages in the systematic review process, highlights that the way we define, extract, assemble, hoard, and process the information stored in primary research influences the stories we tell about our past, current, and future lives (Bowker, 2005). If we hope to help athletes with their performances, increase exercisers' happiness and health, or contribute to the betterment of society, then there is value in considering the way we create the narratives we produce, ensuring we are using suitable storytelling methods that will result in tales worthy of being told and retold. In this chapter, I detail differences between analysis and synthesis, outline factors to help select suitable data analysis and synthesis devices, present a generic set of procedures, and describe a range of specific methods.

What Is Data Analysis and Synthesis?

The Oxford English dictionary defines *analysis* as the "detailed examination of the elements or structure of something." Systematic reviews frequently contain evidence tables summarizing elements from primary research, such as study purpose, sample, method, design features, and results (see ▶ Chapter 7). Evidence tables are outputs from the analysis of primary research. Analysis is a necessary, but often insufficient, systematic review component. If investigators only present an analysis, then readers may be left wondering what the review reveals about the topic and how the project advances knowledge. After analysis, reviewers hoping to make a significant contribution to knowledge may need to engage in data synthesis.

Returning to the Oxford English dictionary, *synthesis* refers to the "combination of components or elements to form a connected whole." Having examined the elements in primary research, reviewers attempt to identify how the studies fit together to provide new knowledge or ways of understanding. For example, a meta-analysis generates a summary effect size for a relationship or variable that represents the best estimate based on existing evidence, along with insight into its precision. Synthesis may involve comparing and contrasting the primary studies: In what ways are they similar and dissimilar? Presenting the results of data synthesis helps answer many questions prominent in readers' minds: What does this all mean? How does it answer the question? (The discussion section in a systematic review is where readers will ask additional questions: How does this advance knowledge? Why should we care?) There is a smorgasbord of ways to analyse and synthesize data, and reviewers face the challenge of selecting a method coherent with their project's purpose.

Selecting a Method

Just as there are many roads leading to Rome, there are several ways to answer a review question. Rome, however, is large, and if you and a friend take alternative roads, you might end up in different parts of the city. Similarly, although there are multiple ways to analyse and synthesize data, they typically do not yield similar answers. In both travelling to Rome and processing systematic review data, useful outcomes result from considering the desired endpoints and the logistics involved in the journey.

To assist in selecting suitable synthesis methods, investigators can reflect on various dimensions that help frame review projects (see ◘ Table 9.1, Gough & Thomas, 2017). Comparing a meta-analysis with a meta-narrative illustrates how the dimensions can assist reviewers in selecting suitable methods.

◘ **Table 9.1** Framing a review project

	Question	
Open	↔	Closed
	Constructs	
Emergent	↔	Predetermined
	Procedures	
Less formal and iterative	↔	Formal and linear
	Inference	
Theoretical	↔	Statistical
	Purpose	
Enlightenment Theory generation	↔	Technical Theory testing

Note Information from Gough and Thomas (2017)

The questions in meta-analyses are generally closed with constructs having been pre-determined and operationally defined. For example, "in the depth jump exercise, how strong is the relationship between box height and jump height?" The reviewers in this example are likely to follow a clear set of formalized procedures to aggregate effect sizes (e.g., correlations) from existing evidence and the project will probably proceed in a linear, stage-like, fashion. They will use statistical estimation on which to base their inferences and meta-analyses are generally designed to test theory in a deductive manner.

During meta-narratives, reviewers describe how lines of research within a topic have evolved over time and the plotlines that explain the constructs, theories, and methods within that body of work (Greenhalgh et al., 2005). The questions in meta-narratives are typically open with constructs being free to emerge and change. For example, sport psychologists have published over the past 30 years numerous reflections on their attempts to help athletes. In a meta-narrative, reviewers will likely pose an open question, such as "what genres and plotlines underlie the articles?" The reviewers will let constructs emerge from, rather than impose them on, the literature. The procedures will be less formal and the reviewers will move back and forth among the search, analysis, synthesis, and interpretation phases. The findings are inferred on theoretical grounds and attention is given to generating new configurations of the evidence.

Different, sometimes conflicting, opinions and practices exist regarding many aspects of the systematic review process, including data analysis and synthesis. Gough and Thomas' (2017) dimensions assist reviewers in establishing strong defences for their methods. According to Stephen King (2000, p. 50): "if you write (or paint or dance or sculpt or sing, I suppose), someone will try to make you feel lousy about it." King's point is echoed in the publication peer review process. The role of peer reviewers is to evaluate the manuscript's originality, contribution, and rigour, often leading to critical and sometimes negative comments. Being able to justify the synthesis methods selected allows you to counter critical comments.

A Generic Set of Analysis and Synthesis Procedures

Authors can select from a range of analysis and synthesis methods. Tables 1.1 and 1.2 from ▶ Chapter 1 presented examples. The myriad of analysis and synthesis practices vary in the breadth of their coverage. Some methods, such as meta-analyses and thematic summaries, focus specifically on data manipulation. Other procedures, such as meta-narratives, realist syntheses, and meta-studies, present broader guidelines that also address other components of the review, such as literature searching and critical appraisal. Referring back to Rome, although each method provides individuals with a different vehicle by which to travel, they are all confined to staying on the same roads. Each method attempts to organize, describe, and combine the information in ways that present a map of the evidence.

The generic process below distinguishes common from specific factors. Different methods have specific factors, often associated with their primary aim. Meta-analyses, for example, use statistical procedures to estimate and explain heterogeneity in a set of effect sizes. Meta-narratives employ literary devices to understand and explain plotlines running through a body of work. Although specific factors separate them, the various methods also share common features, such as: (a) relying on literature generated from a transparent rigorous search; (b) examining the elements, structure, and quality of the evidence; and (c) identifying the meaningfulness and implications of the primary research. The generic process is not designed to replace specific methods, but to help reviewers consider how particular analysis and synthesis procedures (e.g., meta-analysis, meta-narrative) fit within their reviews.

Initial Analysis: Organisation and Description

The first step involves evidence tables and mapping techniques to organize and describe data, giving reviewers an understanding of the primary research. At this point, a systematic map may be sufficient to answer the question and the project can be written up and delivered to stakeholders or published. Often, however, systematic maps are launch pads for deeper analysis and synthesis. During the second stage, investigators use tools to help them analyse and synthesize the primary research to generate answers to sophisticated or tailored questions.

Evidence tables and systematic maps were introduced in ▶ Chapter 7, and form a link between data extraction and analysis. The two methods provide a way to organize the large volume of data that is created during extraction and allow reviewers to track their progress. Evidence tables, for example, help authors identify the elements and structure of each primary study. Systematic maps assist reviewers in describing the body of work as they paint a picture representing the evidence landscape. Together, evidence tables and systematic maps achieve the goals of the initial analysis: organization and description. Having achieved these initial objectives, reviewers are then able to engage in further (and deeper) analysis and synthesis.

Further Analysis and Synthesis

Many textbooks differentiate between quantitative and qualitative review approaches, but the separation sometimes lacks clarity (Thomas, O'Mara-Eves, Harden, & Newman, 2017). Do these labels refer to the primary research, the review methods, or resultant findings? Such a presentation also falsely implies qualitative and quantitative methods are mutually exclusive (Sparkes & Smith, 2014). It is possible, for instance, to generate quantitative findings from qualitative themes and vice versa.

The aggregative/configural continuum discussed in ▶ Chapter 4 provides a way to classify different analysis and synthesis methods. Configurative reviews assemble the evidence, piecing it together to form an answer to the project's question, and often focus on theory development. They strive to explore and interpret data in new ways, often from heterogeneous primary research. Aggregative reviews involve stacking or adding together findings from research, typically to test theory. Data is normally collated from homogenous studies, to gain greater precision and confidence in the findings. The following sections describe ways reviewers can further analyse and synthesize data. These methods are not the only examples, but present some of the common methods in sport, exercise, and physical activity research.

Aggregative Approaches to Synthesis

Vote counting   One common approach to quantitative synthesis is vote counting, usually in relation to significance testing. At the simplest level, researchers count the number of significant versus non-significant findings and decide in favour of the highest frequency. Reviewers may also separate positive from negative significant findings. For example, when examining the effect of a teaching strategy on skill execution, researchers might group a series of studies ($N = 18$) into those where performance changes (a) were non-significant ($n = 6$), (b) indicated significant improvement ($n = 9$), or (c) yielded a significant decrement ($n = 3$). Based on frequencies, the researchers would conclude the teaching strategy increases skill execution. Although seemingly democratic and objective, vote counting has noteworthy limitations (Borenstein, Hedges, Higgins, & Rothstein, 2009; Petticrew & Roberts, 2006).

An underlying assumption is that non-significant findings reveal no effect. Non-significant results, however, might also emerge when an effect is present, but the statistical test is underpowered (Borenstein et al., 2009), a pervasive issue in sport and exercise science research due to small sample sizes (Speed & Andersen, 2000). In such cases, the suitable conclusion is not that there is no effect, but that more research is needed. A further limitation with vote counting is the decision rule to base conclusions on the highest frequency, which could have been as low as 34% in the above teaching strategy example. Some investigators might stipulate that a minimum percentage is needed before concluding that an effect is present. Any decision rule, however, is subjective, and arbitrary changes in the minimum frequency can influence scientific progress and credibility (Hedges & Olkin, 1980).

In addition, vote counting generally disregards heterogeneity among studies and may combine investigations of different quality and design (Light & Smith, 1971; Petticrew & Roberts, 2006). To illustrate, investigators may combine qualitative and quantitative studies, conveniently ignoring that these approaches answer different types of questions. They also overlook that qualitative studies do not allow an inference of statistical significance. Further, vote counting reduces review findings a binary (or ternary) decision. Estimating an effect's magnitude and precision often advances knowledge more than simple yes, no, or maybe responses (Cumming, 2012). Given vote counting's limitations, it is best avoided. If used, however, authors need to acknowledge the limitations involved and explain why they did not employ other, likely more suitable, methods.

Meta-analysis   A meta-analysis involves the statistical pooling of results from a body of research to provide insights into an effect size (Card, 2012). An effect size is "the amount of something that might be of interest" (Cumming, 2012, p. 34), highlighting that meta-analyses are not restricted to examining mean differences between groups in randomized controlled trials. Any numerical variable can be meta-analysed, such as correlations, test reliability estimates, regression coefficients, or even sample characteristics (e.g., mean height, weight, and body mass index). Meta-analyses focus on the results from multiple studies, not the raw data. There are several advantages to undertaking a meta-analysis over other ways of synthesizing quantitative research:

- There is a reduction in reviewer bias (Cooper & Rosenthal, 1980). Reviewers undertaking black box or narrative reviews of quantitative research, for example, can be influenced by superficial properties of the primary research, such as the wording or presentation of information (Bushman & Wells, 2001).
- Meta-analyses often have higher levels of statistical power to detect effects than individual primary research, a useful benefit when the original studies have been based on small sample sizes (Borenstein et al., 2009).
- Meta-analyses typically yield the best estimates of an effect's direction, magnitude, and precision if based on all the available evidence (Cumming, 2012).
- Investigators can evaluate if the variation among primary studies may be attributed to chance or systematic differences between investigations (Petticrew & Roberts, 2006).

Despite the advantages, several criticisms have been levelled at meta-analysis procedures, sometimes laced with humour as illustrated in the journal article titles, *An exercise in meta-silliness* (Eysenck, 1978) and *Meta-analysis/shemata analysis* (Shapiro, 1994). Feinstein (1995, p. 71) described meta-analysis as "statistical alchemy for the 21st century." Common criticisms argue that:

- Meta-analysis involves the mixing of dissimilar studies.
- The inclusion of poorly designed studies invalidates results.
- Important or unpublished studies are disregarded.
- A single numerical estimate does not represent an area of interest adequately.

These criticisms, however, reflect the application of the techniques rather than procedures themselves. For example, critics suggest meta-analysts mix "apples and oranges" or include dissimilar studies yielding meaningless effect size estimates. Exact replication is rare, however, and studies will differ in their characteristics in almost any set of investigations. The decision regarding similarity involves a judgement over which people will have alternative opinions (Borenstein et al., 2009). The argument against mixing dissimilar studies may be reasonable "if apples and oranges are of intrinsic interest on their own, but may not be if they are used to contribute to a wider question about fruit" (Deeks, Higgins, & Altman, 2017, p. 34).

Additionally, the above criticisms are not unique to meta-analysis. The quality of any review, for example, is threatened if authors have not systematically searched the literature to identify the available evidence. Along a similar vein, the inclusion of poor quality studies also threatens both meta-analyses and other review types. Regardless of the synthesis procedures adopted, authors who examine the influence study quality has on their review findings encourage confidence in their conclusions. One helpful feature of meta-analysis procedures is they provide ways to assess the influence of publication (and other types of) bias and study quality on effect size estimates.

The criticism that a single estimate cannot encapsulate a field of study signals a misunderstanding of what meta-analyses are designed to achieve (Borenstein et al., 2009). Meta-analyses, for example, estimate the direction, magnitude, and precision of an effect. It is the role of researchers to interpret the meaningfulness of the estimate, perhaps by considering the variation of effect sizes across the body of work.

If there is a wide range of effect sizes, then reviewers may focus on the dispersion rather than the summary point estimate. If there is a narrow range of effect sizes then readers can have confidence in the robustness of the estimate across the studies (Borenstein et al., 2009).

Thematic summaries   The thematic summary approach reveals that aggregative reviews are not confined to quantitative research, but can also be applied to qualitative investigations. These reviews might be characterized as involving analysis without synthesis. When viewed according to Gough and Thomas' (2017) dimensions in ◻ Table 9.1, these reviews typically ask closed questions focused on pre-specified constructs, such as "what are the sources of stress identified by competitive athletes?" Analysis may follow a pre-determined formal method, such as an adaption of Braun and Clarke's (2013) thematic content analysis procedure originally designed for primary data. Authors may couch their review findings as exploratory and be cautious in identifying applied implications.

Many articles in this genre present an evidence table supplemented with a narrative summary that often does little more than describe the information in the table. There may be no systematic map or attempts to further synthesize the data. Readers are left to infer the meaningfulness of the review findings and generate possible applied implications.

Although thematic summaries can provide useful information, some authors get caught in the traps levelled at vote-counting reviews. To illustrate, there is a tendency to engage in arbitrary counting, such as interpreting a theme as important or meaningful because it appears more often than others. Frequency does not necessarily equate to importance or meaningfulness, however (Krane, Andersen, & Strean, 1997). Findings that seldom appear in the research may be meaningful, but lack visibility for various social, political, or methodological reasons. Without adequate critical thought, thematic summaries may misrepresent primary research.

Configural Approaches to Synthesis

Meta-narrative   The meta-narrative review method is designed for areas that different groups of researchers have conceptualized and studied in separate ways (Greenhalgh et al., 2005). For example, investigators have defined and examined doping in sport from physiological, psychological, sociological, economic, philosophical, and other perspectives. To review doping in ways respectful of each research tradition, we would ask how each group or discipline conceptualized the area, what dimensions they investigated, how they undertook their studies, the justifications for their decisions, and the resulting knowledge (Wong, Greenhalgh, Westhorp, Buckingham, & Pawson, 2013). Different research traditions represent meta-narratives or storylines that give insight into how avenues of scientific inquiry have unfolded over time. A meta-narrative seeks to identify these storylines and bridge them through the discovery of any over-arching narratives. Through meta-narratives, reviewers highlight the contributions of different traditions and what these groups might learn from each other. Kuhn's (1962) book, *The Structure of Scientific Revolutions*, inspired the development of the meta-narrative method. According to Kuhn, science advances in paradigm waves, and that as one tradition gives way to another, yesterday's knowledge, assumptions, and practices become obsolete. In many areas, however, a tradition's knowledge, assumptions, and practices do not necessarily become outdated, but may add to a broader and deeper understanding of the topic area. Given the complexity of many challenges facing people, communities, and societies, teams of researchers from various traditions are more likely to provide sustainable solutions than if working alone. Meta-narratives can provide knowledge and insights to help guide the integration and contribution of multidisciplinary teams.

Although the phases in a meta-narrative mirror those in other analysis practices, including planning, searching, mapping, appraisal, synthesis, and recommendations, the process is not linear, but cyclical with primary research sometimes being double handled as reviewers consider evidence both within its parent tradition and across perspectives (Greenhalgh et al., 2005). As a further similarity with other qualitative and multimethod review frameworks, meta-narratives involve subjective and interpretative decision-making. Researchers, however, make their subjectivity and biases explicit and transparent so that meta-narratives do not become black box reviews. Training materials are freely available online to assist individuals wishing to adopt the framework (▶ http://www.ramesesproject.org/).

Timpka et al. (2015) recently identified three injury and ill health reporting narratives in the sports epidemiology literature: sport performance, clinical examination, and athlete self-report. The performance narrative focused on incapacitation or the impact that injury and illness had on athletes' abilities to participate in their sports. The clinical examination narrative dealt with the influence of sport participation on athlete health, functioning, and well-being. The self-report narrative concentrated on the suitability of athletes' reporting of injury and illness for monitoring purposes. Timpka et al. revealed that parallel reporting practices occurred in the literature. Understanding the different practices assists the comparison and synthesis of studies located within the different narratives.

Realist synthesis   Realist syntheses arose from the need to review evidence regarding complex social and health-related interventions (Pawson, Greenhalgh, Harvey, & Walshe, 2004), although they can also guide the synthesis of knowledge about other multifarious phenomena. Similar to most other systematic review methods, realist syntheses are not limited to reviewing experimental research. Many challenges in sport, exercise, and physical activity contexts necessitate the amalgamation of studies of various designs across several disciplines. Given the heterogeneity of the research and complexity of topics, linear aggregative review procedures are often inadequate to provide integrated and useful information. Sport psychologist training is an example. There is no universal training pathway because globally, and even within countries, educational programmes vary considerably, even if regulated by professional bodies. It makes little sense to examine if sport psychologist training works, because there is no gold standard or discrete intervention to examine. Instead, useful knowledge results from identifying what types of educational experiences are helpful for which types of trainees, why are they helpful, and under what circumstances. Flexible and innovative review methods are needed to integrate disparate sources of relevant knowledge.

Reviewers conducting realist syntheses do not focus, typically, on specific interventions, because they are seldom, if ever, replicated exactly across contexts. Instead, interventions are prone to modification because they represent open systems and include people who respond to micro and macro feedback loops (Pawson et al., 2004). Realist syntheses evaluate underlying programme theories describing participants' actions and interactions. Further, programme theories detail nonlinear process chains that involve context, mechanisms, and outputs and are embedded within social environments. A process chain in sport psychologist training details that testing a psychological strategy (mechanism) during a placement (context) allows students to learn how to adapt interventions to fit athletes' needs (output).

Yen, Flood, Thompson, Anderson, and Wong (2014) conducted a realist synthesis examining how characteristics of built environments influence older adults' decisions about physical activity. They proposed an initial ecological programme theory that considers mobility to be a function of the individual, the environment, and the interactions among people and their surroundings. The literature search located 123 studies of various designs and focused on a range of built environments. The revised programme theory contained process chains centred on perceptions of safety (traffic and crime). Specifically, aesthetics (the appeal of the surroundings), land use (residential, commercial, public), and connectivity (intersections, sidewalks, street networks) emerged as key external contextual factors, along with cognitive and physical capacity as internal contextual variables, that shaped decisions about mobility (output), primarily through perceptions of safety (mechanisms). Yen et al.'s synthesis provides guidance for supporting older adult's physical activity: they need to perceive it is safe for them to be mobile. Further, the synthesis revealed aspects of the built environment that could be adapted to encourage perceptions of safety, including aesthetics, land use, and connectivity.

Mixed Method Reviews

Research producers and consumers recognize that perfect studies do not exist, and the overwhelming majority make incremental rather than earth-shattering advances in knowledge. Single studies typically do not provide complete solutions to the problems facing communities. Along with the diversification of research designs in sport, exercise, and physical activity, stakeholders have become interested in mixed method projects to allow greater insights into the challenges and problems in modern societies. In turn, there has been increasing interest in mixed method reviews.

A common definition of mixed method reviews is that they combine qualitative and quantitative research, but this seemingly obvious description is misleading. First, qualitative and quantitative designs ask different questions. For example, if a quantitative study showed a positive relationship between two variables, and a qualitative investigation found that people perceive an association, it is not meaningful to conclude there are multiple studies indicating a link. The suitable conclusion is that one study reveals a correlation and another shows that people believe a link exists. Second, the definition is typically applied to the mixing of quantitative and qualitative research, but it is also relevant to the blending of studies within the same broad church. For example, there are several schools of qualitative research (e.g., grounded theory, narrative analysis, phenomenology, etc.), yet people may naively assume the findings from separate approaches can be combined despite their different foci and methods. If authors do not consider the theoretical or methodological underpinning of the primary research, then their reviews may provide misleading interpretations. Some factors to address when considering a mixed method review include coherence, sequencing, emphasis, and guiding theory (Creswell, 2014; Thomas et al., 2017).

Coherence Establishing the coherence among the review question, primary research design, and extracted data helps determine if and how to engage in a mixed method review. For example, if the review is focused on a question regarding an intervention's efficacy then experimental research generating standardized numerical pre- and post-test data is suitable for inclusion. If the focus is on how people story their experience with the intervention then a narrative approach that identifies the genres and plot arcs underlying their accounts is warranted. These example review questions are singular in focus, and may be addressed with one type of research. Multimethod reviews are suitable for projects addressing a cluster or series of interrelated questions, such as why does the intervention work, for whom, and in what circumstances (Petticrew & Roberts, 2006)?

Timing or sequencing Reviewers have a range of sequencing options and they may select one that suits the project's purpose and development (Pluye & Hong, 2014; Creswell, 2014). Sequential designs include undertaking separate reviews that focus on specific interrelated questions, but together tell a broader story. For example, a qualitative review is conducted first to identify relevant effective coach characteristics favoured by athletes, followed by a quantitative synthesis to establish how those attributes vary with coaching level. Alternatively, a quantitative review might focus on attribute variation first, and then a qualitative review might shed light on how those characteristics express themselves in particular contexts.

Parallel reviews occur at the same time (if the review team is large enough) and emerge from the initial systematic map. For example, a team might start by mapping the research associated with a topic and then identify two or more specific narrower questions worthy of further exploration. The team might then present these sub-projects separately or may engage in a higher order synthesis to bring the individual reviews together. A convergent approach involves bringing the different types of primary research together in one synthesis, but often involves the transformation of data, such as turning qualitative data into numbers, or finding ways to amalgamate quantitative data to represent a qualitative pattern or theme (Creswell, 2014). Less agreement exists among reviewers regarding the feasibility of convergent approaches. For example, although some individuals equate the presence of a theme in a qualitative study with a significant result from a quantitative study and include both in a vote counting review, other people highlight the conceptual and methodological shortcomings of the practice.

Weighting or emphasis of each component   Reviewers might need to consider the weight they give to each type of data or review method (Creswell, 2014). They may, for example, treat each component equally or delegate one a supportive role in the overall project. Decisions about weighting or emphasis are influenced by the reviewers' and intended audience's preferences. For example, policymakers may want primarily to know the efficacy of an intervention (a quantitative question). They may also wish to have enough insight into people's experiences of the intervention so they can appreciate ways it is received. Practitioners, however, may have greater interest in the qualitative component of the previous example than the quantitative aspect, because they want to determine how best to work with people getting the intervention. Establishing the preferred emphasis to give each aspect of a mixed method review helps with the allocation of time, labour, and resources.

Guiding theory   Another consideration when deciding if and how to undertake a mixed method review is your theoretical framework. Recall from ▶ Chapter 3 that a theoretical framework describes your understanding of the content area and underlying knowledge assumptions. Theoretical frameworks help when deciding what questions are worth asking, which methods are relevant, and in what ways do different questions and methods complement and differ from each other. Answers to these questions vary among people and carry implications for what can or cannot be achieved in a review. Although some people, for example, think qualitative studies can be combined meaningfully, others disagree because doing so decontextualizes the findings (Petticrew & Roberts, 2006). Turning to a quantitative example, opinion varies regarding whether experimental and descriptive data can be synthesized in the same project.

Mixed method review checklist   There exist a number of tools to help people plan, conduct, or evaluate systematic reviews. The majority of these are focused on single method rather than mixed method reviews. Although not tailored to mixed method reviews, they still help authors and audiences assess the strengths and weaknesses of the project. The items in ◘ Table 9.2 are adapted from Creswell's

◘ **Table 9.2**	Questions to assist mixed method review design
1	Is a definition of the mixed method review design included?
2	Do the review purposes suit a mixed method approach?
3	Is it explained how the review will advance knowledge?
4	Will the review have a real world impact?
5	Have the criteria for selecting the specific methods been given?
6	Is there coherence across review questions, methods, analysis, and synthesis?
7	Is the overall review structure detailed (perhaps featuring a flowchart)?
8	Have each of the individual methods been adequately explained?
9	Has the procedure for review synthesis been addressed?
10	Are the criteria for assessing the review quality explicit?

(2014) list of questions to help evaluate mixed method research to suit a mixed method review. These questions can complement other evaluation tools such as AMSTAR-2 (▶ https://amstar.ca/) or the CASP checklist (▶ https://casp-uk.net/).

Chapter Case Example: What Are the Barriers and Facilitators of Children's Fruit and Vegetable Consumption?

Thomas et al.'s (2003) review investigating the barriers to, and facilitators of, children's (aged 4–10 years old) consumption of fruit and vegetables illustrates how mixed method reviews can contribute to knowledge and social policy. The report is freely available from the EPPI-Centre (▶ https://eppi.ioe. ac.uk). After mapping, scoping, and stakeholder consultation exercises, the authors undertook two reviews before combing the findings of each to generate new knowledge and recommendations. The two reviews included a meta-analysis of controlled trials to assess intervention effectiveness and a thematic synthesis of qualitative studies exploring children's views on food and healthy eating.

The meta-analysis revealed that collectively a range of interventions increased daily consumption of fruit by a fifth of a portion, and vegetables by almost a fifth. Effects varied and were larger, for example, in interventions targeted at parents with cardiovascular disease risk factors and those which did not dilute a fruit and vegetable message by promoting other lifestyle changes. Single component interventions were ineffective.

The thematic synthesis yielded insights into children's perspectives. Results, for instance, suggested that children (a) do not believe it is their role to be interested in health; (b) do not perceive messages about future health as personally relevant or credible; (c) ascribe different meanings to fruit, vegetables, and confectionery; (d) desire control over their food choices; (e) value social eating; and (f) observe contradictions between what is promoted and what adults provide. These themes underpinned implications for suitable interventions, including promoting fruit and vegetables as tasty rather than healthy, making health messages relevant to children, and allowing them ownership of their food choices.

To combine the two sets of studies, Thomas et al. (2003) compared the interventions to the nine implications from the qualitative studies. If a sufficient number of studies existed, the authors conducted a meta-analysis to compare interventions with components matching the implications with those without a match. Interventions with components matching children's views were either clearly effective or unclear in their effects, but none were ineffective or harmful. Those interventions with larger effect sizes had at least one of the components matching children's views, including: (a) the promotion of fruit and vegetables in separate interventions or in different ways within the same intervention; (b) a reduction in the emphasis on health messages; and (c) the promotion of fruit and vegetables in educational materials accompanied by access to fruit and vegetables. The effectiveness of interventions with the following components, however, was unclear: branding fruit and vegetables as exciting or child-friendly, and encouraging children to express choice. Gaps between interventions and children's views revealed opportunities for innovative strategies, such as: branding fruit and vegetables as tasty, and not healthy; allowing children influence over the context in which they eat; and making health messages credible.

Summary

Stories describe real or imaginary people and events. Authors tell stories for various purposes, including entertainment, enlightenment, or expression, and stories belong to different genres. Systematic reviews are a genre aiming to reflect our understanding of some phenomenon or topic of interest. Some systematic review stories hope to capture an accurate representation of the way the world is, whereas others offer one possibility, as perceived by the authors, of many potential views of reality. Nonfiction storytelling is a difficult craft to master, and the ability to weave threads of evidence and lines of argument together emerges only from diligent practice. My purpose in the current chapter has been to illustrate possible ways to analyse and synthesize primary research evidence to help investigators write systematic review tales that provide answers to their questions, and do more than clutter dusty library shelves or tie up computer hard disk memory. Having constructed answers to review questions, authors are ready to assess the adequacy of the new knowledge, the focus of the next chapter.

9

❓ Learning Exercises

1. Develop a table that summarizes the various specific approaches to data analysis and synthesis that you could use to help you select methods in future reviews (you can use those listed in this chapter, those in ► Chapter 1, and those from other sources). Each row represents a method, such as meta-analysis, realist synthesis, meta-study, etc. In the column headings place Gough and Thomas' (2017) considerations as illustrated in ◘ Table 9.1: questions, constructs, procedures, inferences, and purpose. For each cell provide a short description of how the method deals with the consideration.

2. Review the analysis and synthesis strategy you presented in your proposal from ► Chapter 2. Modify it in light of the current chapter so that there is optimal coherence between the question and answer.

References

Borenstein, M., Hedges, L. V., Higgins, J. P. T., & Rothstein, H. R. (2009). *Introduction to meta-analysis*. Chichester, UK: Wiley.

Bowker, G. C. (2005). *Memory practices in the sciences*. Cambridge: MIT Press.

Braun, V., & Clarke, V. (2013). *Successful qualitative research: A practical guide for beginners*. Thousand Oaks, CA.: Sage.

Bushman, B. J., & Wells, G. L. (2001). Narrative impressions of literature: The availability bias and the corrective properties of meta-analytic approaches. *Personality and Social Psychology Bulletin, 27*, 1123–1130. ► https://doi.org/10.1177/0146167201279005.

Card, N. A. (2012). *Applied meta-analysis for social science research*. New York, NY: Guilford.

Cooper, H. M., & Rosenthal, R. (1980). Statistical versus traditional procedures for summarizing research findings. *Psychological Bulletin, 87*, 442–449. ► https://doi.org/10.1037/0033-2909.87.3.442.

Creswell, J. W. (2014). *Research design: Qualitative, quantitative, and mixed methods approaches* (4th ed.). Thousand Oaks, CA: Sage.

Cumming, G. (2012). *Understanding the new statistics: Effect sizes, confidence intervals, and meta-analysis*. New York, NY: Routledge.

Deeks, J. J., Higgins, J. P. T., & Altman, D. G. (2017). Analysing data and undertaking meta-analyses. In J. P. T. Higgins, R. Churchill, J. Chandler, & M. S. Cumpston (Eds.), *Cochrane handbook for systematic reviews of interventions* (version 5.2.0). Retrieved from ▶ www.training.cochrane.org/handbook.

Eysenck, H. J. (1978). An exercise in mega-silliness. *American Psychologist, 33,* 517. ▶ https://doi.org/10.1037/0003-066X.33.5.517.a.

Feinstein, A. R. (1995). Meta-analysis: Statistical alchemy for the 21st century. *Journal of Clinical Epidemiology, 48,* 71–79. ▶ https://doi.org/10.1016/0895-4356(94)00110-C.

Gough, D., & Thomas, J. (2017). Commonality and diversity in reviews. In D. Gough, S. Oliver, & J. Thomas (Eds.), *An introduction to systematic reviews* (2nd ed., pp. 43–70). Thousand Oaks, CA: Sage.

Greenhalgh, T., Robert, G., Macfarlane, F., Bate, P., Kyriakidou, O., & Peacock, R. (2005). Storylines of research in diffusion of innovation: A meta-narrative approach to systematic review. *Social Science and Medicine, 61,* 417–430. ▶ https://doi.org/10.1016/j.socscimed.2004.12.001.

Hedges, L. V., & Olkin, I. (1980). Vote-counting methods in research synthesis. *Psychological Bulletin, 88,* 359–369. ▶ https://doi.org/10.1037/0033-2909.88.2.359.

King, S. (2000). *On writing: A memoir of the craft*. New York, NY: Scribner.

Krane, V., Andersen, M. B., & Strean, W. B. (1997). Issues of qualitative research methods and presentation. *Journal of Sport and Exercise Psychology, 19,* 213–218. ▶ https://doi.org/10.1123/jsep.19.2.213.

Kuhn, T. S. (1962). *The structure of scientific revolutions*. Chicago, IL: University of Chicago.

Light, R., & Smith, P. (1971). Accumulating evidence: Procedures for resolving contradictions among different research studies. *Harvard Educational Review, 41,* 429–471. ▶ https://doi.org/10.17763/haer.41.4.437714870334w144.

Pawson, R., Greenhalgh, T., Harvey, G., & Walshe, K. (2004). *Realist synthesis: An introduction*. Manchester, UK: Economic and Social Research Council.

Petticrew, M., & Roberts, H. (2006). *Systematic reviews in the social sciences: A practical guide*. Malden, MA: Blackwell.

Pluye, P., & Hong, Q. N. (2014). Combining the power of stories and the power of numbers: Mixed methods research and mixed studies reviews. *Annual Review of Public Health, 35,* 29–45. ▶ https://doi.org/10.1146/annurev-publhealth-032013-182440.

Shapiro, S. (1994). Meta-analysis/shmeta-analysis. *American Journal of Epidemiology, 140,* 771–778. ▶ https://doi.org/10.1093/oxfordjournals.aje.a117324.

Sparkes, A. C., & Smith, B. (2014). *Qualiative research methods in sport, exercise, and health: From process to product*. Abingdon, OX: Routledge.

Speed, H. D., & Andersen, M. B. (2000). What exercise and sport scientists don't understand. *Journal of Science and Medicine in Sport, 3,* 84–92. ▶ https://doi.org/10.1016/S1440-2440(00)80051-1.

Thomas, J., O'Mara-Eves, A., Harden, A., & Newman, M. (2017). Synthesis methods for combining and configuring textual or mixed methods data. In D. Gough, S. Oliver, & J. Thomas (Eds.), *An introduction to systematic reviews* (2nd ed., pp. 181–209). Thousand Oaks: Sage.

Thomas, J., Sutcliffe, K., Harden, A., Oakley, A., Oliver, S., Rees, R., … Kavanagh, J. (2003). *Children and healthy eating: A systematic review of barriers and facilitators*. London, UK: EPPI-Centre, Social Science Research Unit, Institute of Education, University of London.

Timpka, T., Jacobsson, J., Ekberg, J., Finch, C. F., Bichenbach, J., Edouard, P., … Alonso, J. M. (2015). Meta-narrative analysis of sports injury reporting practices based on the Injury Definitions Concept Framework (IDCF): A review of consensus statements and epidemiological studies in athletics (track and field). *Journal of Science and Medicine in Sport, 18,* 643–650. ▶ https://doi.org/10.1016/j.jsams.2014.11.393.

Wong, G., Greenhalgh, T., Westhorp, G., Buckingham, J., & Pawson, R. (2013). RAMESES publication standards: Meta-narrative reviews. *BMC Medicine, 11,* article 20. ▶ https://doi.org/10.1186/1741-7015-11-20.

Yen, I. H., Fandel Flood, J., Thompson, H., Anderson, L. A., & Wong, G. (2014). How design of places promotes or inhibits mobility of older adults: Realist synthesis of 20 years of research. *Journal of Aging and Health, 26,* 1340–1372. ▶ https://doi.org/10.1177/0898264314527610.

Assessing the Systematic Review

D. Tod, *Conducting Systematic Reviews in Sport, Exercise, and Physical Activity*,
https://doi.org/10.1007/978-3-030-12263-8_10

Learning Outcomes

After reading this chapter, you should be able to:
- Describe the reasons for assessing a systematic review.
- Identify criteria to help evaluate a systematic review.
- Detail the GRADE procedures.
- Develop criteria for assessing configural reviews of qualitative research.

Introduction

The following story is a Persian fable featuring the character Nasrudin, a popular figure among Sufi teachers (Shah, 1966):

» Someone saw Nasrudin searching for something on the ground under a street light.
"What have you lost, Mulla?" he asked.
"My key," said the Mulla. So they both went down on their knees and looked for it.
After a time the other man asked: "Where exactly did you drop it?"
"In my own house."
"Then why are you looking here?"
"There is more light here than inside my own house."

10

Nasrudin's mistake was looking in the wrong location, but there are other ways he might have hindered his ability to find his key. For example, if Nasrudin had employed a torch but not known how to use it, then it would not have worked correctly, causing him to miss his key. If Nasrudin was not looking for his key, but needed light for another purpose, then a normal light or torch may not have been helpful. For example, if he was verifying the authenticity of a British £10 note, Nasrudin would have been better served with an ultra-violet light source. These are three ways his search may have been stymied: looking in the wrong location, not using the equipment properly, and using an irrelevant tool.

Each of the above three mistakes highlight ways that systematic reviews can lose credibility with readers and point to criteria by which we can evaluate the quality of a project. First, a review can focus on literature stakeholders consider irrelevant (searching in the wrong place). Second, investigators may implement the review method incorrectly (not using equipment properly). Third, investigators might select a review method that is not apt for the question (using an unsuitable method). In this chapter I focus on critically appraising the review (► Chapter 8 discussed assessing the located evidence). Specifically, I address the reasons for evaluating the review, suitable assessment criteria, GRADE procedures for appraising a review's findings, and possible ways to assess configural reviews.

Reasons for Appraising a Review

Several reasons exist for knowing how to evaluate a review. For example, understanding how to assess a review helps investigators plan their work and produce products to the best of their abilities. Once completed, high quality reviews advance knowledge in substantial ways. They also provide insights regarding future avenues of research worthy of exploration.

Further, reviews guide decision-making, policy, and practice. Understanding how confident we can be in the review's findings allows us to use that information wisely to inform how we govern ourselves and our communities. High quality reviews, in medicine for example, save lives. Equally, however, reliance on poor reviews may endanger health and well-being. These consequences are not limited to medicine. The reviews that sport, exercise, and physical activity researchers undertake influence practice and policy in many health-related settings, and projects containing misleading results can lead to detrimental physical, psychological, and perhaps even fatal, consequences.

Even if reviews are focused on topics unlikely to result in loss of life, physical capacity, or mental well-being, it is helpful to remember that people make decisions related to all facets of human involvement in sport, exercise, and physical activity. The better informed they are of the risks, safeguards, benefits, and costs involved, the greater the likelihood they will make decisions ensuring that their own and others' experiences in sport, exercise, and physical activity are positive rather than negative. Systematic reviews can have a significant role in helping people make salubrious decisions.

In addition, poor science can damage the credibility of a discipline. It is in researchers' and practitioners' interests to ensure that the work being disseminated is of the best quality possible. Much has been written about the limitations, weaknesses, and misuses of science (Aronowitz, 1988; Fanelli, 2012; Ioannidis, 2005; Oreskes & Conway, 2010). It is correct that there are limitations to the scientific method, there are questions investigators cannot answer, and there are reasons researchers are tempted to act unscientifically. Nevertheless, it is unhelpful to give easy ammunition to people who are sceptical of research and its benefits.

Criteria for Evaluating a Review

Often, textbooks describing how to do systematic reviews either skirt around or avoid addressing how authors can appraise the quality of their projects. If textbooks do address the issue, they may limit discussion to possible reporting standards authors can follow. Although reporting standards, such as the PRISMA checklist, have a beneficial role, they usually do not address all the relevant aspects in review appraisal. Recently, Liabo, Gough, and Harden (2017) outlined three dimensions to consider when evaluating a systematic synthesis, including the review method, the primary studies, and the resulting evidence summary.

Assessing the Review Method

Three components are involved in evaluating the review method: rigour, suitability, and focus. Each is described below.

Method Rigour

The first dimension refers to the rigour of the method reviewers applied. Multiple reporting standards and methodological checklists exist to guide the assessment of a systematic review's rigour. AMSTAR-2 (A Measurement Tool to Assess Systematic Reviews) is an example designed for reviews containing randomized and non-randomized studies of health care interventions (Shea et al., 2017). There are 16 questions and these are presented in ◨ Table 10.1. Some of the various checklists are generic, whereas others are focused on particular types of reviews, such as the standards for meta-narrative and realist syntheses the RAMESES project has made available (▶ https://www.ramesesproject.org/).

There are limitations with using checklists. Many are well suited to aggregative reviews that follow a predetermined method, but are not always appropriate for iterative projects relying on emergent designs (Liabo et al., 2017). Also, for various reasons, it is not always possible to be completely transparent when reporting a review. There are, for example, space limitations in journals and authors may not be able to articulate reasons behind some of their decisions (Hammersley, 2006). Despite their limitations, checklists have a useful role in the assessment of a review's rigour.

Method Suitability

Investigators may have implemented a review method with care, but selected an approach unable to answer the question. The use of incorrect procedures leads to incoherence between the review's questions and findings, perhaps resulting in the

10

◨ **Table 10.1**   Topics included in AMSTAR-2

Item	Topic
1	Did the review question and inclusion criteria conform to the PICO acronym?
2	Did the report indicate the timing of protocol development and adjustments?
3	Did the review discuss study design as an inclusion criterion?
4	Did the review include a comprehensive search?
5	Did the report indicate duplicated study selection?
6	Did the review indicate duplicated data extraction?
7	Did the review identify and justify excluded studies?
8	Did the report adequately describe included studies?
9	Did the review outline a suitable risk of bias?
10	Did the report identify sources of funding for primary studies?
11	If performed, did the review detail a suitable meta-analysis?
12	If performed, did the meta-analysis assess of the influence of the risk of bias results on review findings?
13	Did the report consider risk of bias when interpreting the review's findings?
14	Did the review explain and discuss heterogeneity?
15	Did the report explore and discuss publication bias?
16	Did the report discuss review author conflict of interests?

report being unable to satisfy stakeholder needs. In recent years, researchers have proposed numerous ways to synthesize qualitative literature and these procedures can appear similar on the surface, so it may not always be easy to select an apt method for a project (Barnett-Page & Thomas, 2009). Normally, however, taking the time to examine the approach or getting advice from its creator by email can help. To illustrate, both framework synthesis and meta-narrative can be applied to the same body of research, but they generate different types of answers. A meta-narrative reveals how a body of research has evolved over time (Greenhalgh et al., 2005), whereas a framework synthesis proposes a conceptual model describing our understanding of the topic area (Oliver et al., 2008). The choice between the two review methods depends on the intended audiences' needs.

Method Focus

The third dimension relates to the choice of primary research (Liabo et al., 2017). Investigators may have selected a suitable method, implemented it correctly, but focused it in a way that reduces coherence between the project's aims, purposes, and procedures. Incoherence, for example, occurs if the primary evidence that investigators reviewed does not reflect the breadth of stakeholder's questions. In strength and conditioning, reviewers might examine studies comparing single- with multiple-set resistance training programmes in beginner lifters to determine which leads to greater strength gains. Strength and conditioning coaches, however, may ask what is the best way to increase strength in beginners? The stakeholder's question is broad and involves much more than just the number of sets, whereas the researcher's focus is narrow. The example illustrates the value of negotiating with stakeholders to ensure clarity regarding aims and methods.

Assessing the Included Studies

In ▶ Chapter 8 I discussed critical appraisal of primary research, and much of the material is relevant for assessing the quality of the review. If the primary research on which a synthesis rests is poor or non-existent, then the review's report card would read "applied well but reveals weak (or no) evidence." Stakeholders can then decide the value of the review for their purposes. The above three dimensions for evaluating a review are also suitable for evaluating the included studies: study method, study suitability, and study focus.

Included Study Rigour

Study rigour refers to the soundness of its method or its internal validity. As discussed in ▶ Chapter 8, there are numerous tools to help reviewers assess the rigour of an individual study although the degree to which these rules can be coded for critical appraisal varies across different designs.

Included Study Design Suitability

Reviewers may select studies that are not relevant to the question. Well-worn examples include the use of descriptive research to imply causality or the use of qualitative investigations to determine a relationship between two variables.

Included Study Focus

Study focus deals with the match between the review question and the findings of primary research. Included studies may have data relevant to the review despite the focus of the primary investigations being generally unsuitable. To illustrate, when meta-analysing findings regarding a relationship between two variables, investigators may extract data from studies where those two variables were only two of a number that were measured for a broader purpose, such as testing a theory.

Appraising the Evidence Synthesis

Liabo et al.'s (2017) third dimension is the evaluation of the extent the review's evidence synthesis answers the question. Whereas dimension two referred to an appraisal of the individual studies in the review, dimension three assesses the findings that emerged from combining the primary research. The two criteria in dimension three include (a) the nature of the body of included studies and (b) the extent of the evidence.

The first criterion considers the coherence or fit of the included studies. In a meta-analysis, for example, it is just as easy to generate a summary effect size from highly heterogeneous studies as from homogeneous investigations. Audiences, however, will have greater confidence in effect sizes from homogeneous studies than from heterogeneous investigations, because the former is more likely based on research examining the same phenomena than the later. In configural reviews, coherence refers to the linkages or relationships among the studies: do they seem plausible or convoluted? Do the arguments and evidence for the synthesis fit together logically or do the authors seem to be speculating and engaging in conceptual sleight of hand to make their points?

The second criterion examines the extent of the evidence. Taken together, the included studies may provide a synthesis that is insufficient in scope or depth to allow an adequate answer to the question. Readers may question the reliability, generalizability, credibility, or trustworthiness of the synthesis to advance knowledge or support decision-making, even though it was based on high quality studies.

The two criteria of fit and extent are not independent of each other. It may be difficult, for example, to provide a coherent answer to a question when there are just a few studies. The greater the number of relevant high quality studies there are, the more likely reviewers can develop a coherent answer to a question. Liabo et al.'s (2017) criteria identify what to assess, but they need to be operationalized. The GRADE system is one way to assess the evidence synthesis and has begun appearing in sport, exercise, and physical activity literature.

Grading of Recommendations Assessment, Development, and Evaluation (GRADE)

The GRADE tool offers a transparent process for developing, presenting, and evaluating evidence summaries generated from systematic reviews. Further, GRADE also helps policymakers develop recommendations based on those reviews (Guyatt et al., 2011). GRADE procedures detail how to frame questions, select and rate the importance of relevant outcomes of interest, evaluate a body of evidence, and combine scientific information with other considerations when developing recommendations. Although the system was designed for healthcare interventions or management strategies, it could be used in other domains, such as sport, exercise, and physical activity.

Review Process

■ Figure 10.1 presents an overview of the GRADE process. The tasks above the horizontal line apply to systematic reviews. The activities below the line relate to policy recommendations. Investigators begin by defining their questions in terms of the PICO acronym. Ideally, the list of outcomes includes all variables relevant to the studied population. Investigators classify these outcomes as either critical or not critical but important.

A systematic search is undertaken to identify relevant studies which are mapped against the outcomes. After data extraction, reviewers estimate the effect sizes and confidence intervals associated with each outcome. GRADE was tailored towards the meta-analysis of quantitative research. Recently GRADE has been

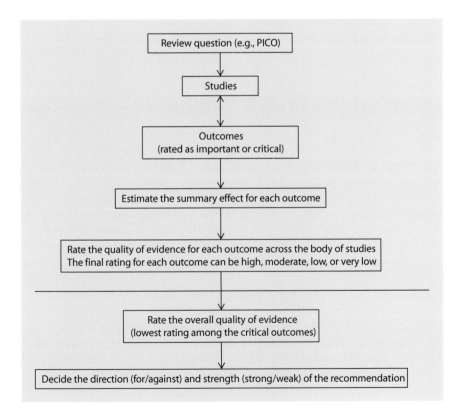

■ **Fig. 10.1**   Overview of the GRADE procedures

modified to help investigators assess findings from a synthesis of qualitative evidence (Lewin et al., 2015).

When assessing quality, GRADE's attention is directed to the body of evidence for each outcome and not individual studies. Each outcome gets an initial quality rating of high, moderate, low, or very low. Ratings are then adjusted according to factors listed below. Outcomes based on randomized controlled trials have an initial rating of high, whereas those underpinned by observational studies start on low. The five factors that lower an initial rating include (Liabo et al., 2017):

- Risk of bias (e.g., randomization).
- Inconsistency across studies (unexplained heterogeneity).
- Indirectness which refers to the applicability of findings to the population of interest (external validity) or absence of direct comparisons between the alternative interventions being compared.
- Imprecision of results (e.g., width of confidence intervals).
- Publication bias.

Ratings may be reduced by one or two levels depending on whether the factor's effect is considered serious or very serious. The three factors that raise an initial rating include:

- Large effect sizes.
- Presence of a dose-response gradient.
- Accounting for plausible confounding variables.

10

Evidence Profile and Summary of Findings

For systematic reviews, GRADE results in an evidence quality rating and an estimate of an effect's direction, magnitude, and precision for each outcome (Guyatt et al., 2011). For example, after a meta-analysis has been conducted on the influence of a physiological training method on an attribute of human performance, the result might indicate (a) an effect size of 0.6 (direction and magnitude), (b) a 95% confidence interval of 0.54–0.66 (precision), and (c) a GRADE quality rating of low (suggesting a lack of confidence in the intervention). The information across outcomes may be presented in one of two tables: an evidence profile or a summary of findings. ◼ Table 10.2 is an example of a summary of findings table generated from a meta-analysis examining the relationship between muscular obsession and exercise and dietary behaviour (results are taken from Tod & Edwards, 2015). A summary of findings table typically records the most pertinent results, provides the quality rating, and may offer comments regarding the quality assessment. Evidence profiles typically provide full details regarding the findings and the quality ratings. Both tables (evidence profile and summary of findings) may also include additional information, such as sample sizes and number of studies. The two tables serve different audiences. Summary of findings tables are for end users who need the key information, whereas evidence profiles are for people wanting to understand the reasons outcomes received particular assigned ratings (Guyatt et al., 2011).

Table 10.2 GRADE summary of findings for muscular obsession and health behaviours

Outcome	No. of studies	ES (95% CI)	Quality rating	Comments
Weight training	15	0.31 (0.21–0.41)	Very low	Observational research, rating dropped due publication bias, high risk of bias, and confounding
Non weight training	24	0.11 (0.01–0.21)	Very low	Observational research, rating dropped due publication bias, high risk of bias, and confounding
Exercise dependence	11	0.43 (0.33–0.53)	Very low	Observational research, rating dropped due publication bias, high risk of bias, and confounding
Disordered eating	49	0.30 (0.26–0.34)	Very low	Observational research, rating dropped due publication bias, high risk of bias, and confounding
Dietary supplement use	16	0.36 (0.26–0.44)	Very low	Observational research, rating dropped due publication bias, high risk of bias, and confounding

Note ES = effect size, 95% CI = 95% confidence interval

Developing Recommendations

As illustrated in ■ Fig. 10.1, after the evidence for each outcome has been graded, recommendation developers make a verdict regarding an overall rating of quality that includes direction and strength. Recommendation direction is influenced by (a) the balance between desirable and undesirable outcomes and (b) patients' values and preferences (in relation to healthcare interventions). Recommendation strength is also influenced by these two factors, plus the quality of the evidence. Both direction and strength evaluations may be adjusted in light of resource use implications.

GRADE treats quality as a series of discrete categories rather than on a continuum (Guyatt et al., 2011). The quality rating is also an amalgamation of several factors, some of which are multidimensional. GRADE does not provide an objective simple quality rating, but represents an overall subjective impression. Although GRADE does not lead to ratings with which everyone will agree, it is a method to help make rating and recommendation production systematic, transparent, and malleable to people's attitudes and preferences (Guyatt et al. 2011).

The GRADE approach was developed for healthcare interventions, policies, and management strategies, not for other topics such as risk identification or diagnosis (Guyatt et al., 2011). Experimental research and randomized controlled trials are privileged over descriptive work, although the GRADE creators recognize that observational studies have some value in assessing healthcare services. The framework is also suited towards aggregative reviews and meta-analyses. These two observations reflect the broader tradition in systematic reviewing, particularly in health domains which have strongly influenced research synthesis in sport, exercise, and physical activity. In recent years, as systematic reviewing methodology has developed and broadened, greater consideration has been directed towards how to evaluate configural reviews of qualitative research.

Evaluating Configural Reviews

The criteria and tools presented so far may be applied to aggregative reviews with greater ease than to configural syntheses, particularly those containing qualitative research. Systematic reviewers and methodologists have great affinity for checklists, crib sheets, and worksheets (Chalmers & Altman, 1995). These tools serve useful purposes, such as directing reviewers' attention towards meaningful questions about quality and helping them to remember details needed to evaluate a project. Also, these tools promote minimum and consistent standards across reviews which assist in lubricating communication among scientists, academics, and stakeholders. From an educational perspective these tools help people new to systematic reviewing to learn how to assess projects.

These quality control tools, however, typically reflect a positivistic or post-positivistic world view that dominates medical, health, sport, exercise, and physical activity research. From this viewpoint, reviewers seek to apply predetermined criteria to evaluate their projects. Such criteria lean towards a belief in an objective reality, out of which universal markers of quality can be invoked. In the absence of a belief of an objective reality, it is difficult to defend universal, predetermined, or standardized checklists that can be applied to all systematic reviews. Some groups recognize the difficulty in justifying all-encompassing tools and tailor their crib sheets to particular types of reviews, such as AMSTAR-2 which is designed for experimental studies. There are reasons why universal predetermined objective criteria may be unsuitable for configural reviews of qualitative research.

Researchers vary in their beliefs that configural reviews provide unblemished windows allowing a view of a single objective reality (Pope, Mays, & Popay, 2007). Some people believe there is no single objective social reality to be viewed through the window. Other individuals think the window is smudged, making it difficult to see the reality on the other side. These individual suggest the window one uses influences what is seen on the other side. If the window influences one's view or if a single objective social reality does not exist, then universal predetermined criteria are unlikely to be suitable for every configural review, because they involve subjective judgements for which there are no right or wrong answers.

In addition, many quality control checklists have not been rigorously tested and evaluated (Liabo et al., 2017). Ironically, although evidence-based practice is a value underpinning systematic reviewing, many tools lack data showing that they are suitable or work as intended. Further, the application of universal criteria may hinder scientific progress if they get applied to innovative and novel ways of reviewing research that are not underpinned by a positivistic or post-positivistic world view.

One Way to Assess Configural Reviews

In recent years, Smith and colleagues have wrestled with how to evaluate the credibility of qualitative research in sport, exercise, and physical activity (Smith & Caddick, 2012; Sparkes & Smith, 2014). They have advocated a relativist approach that can also inform the assessment of configural reviews in the area. A starting point is the suggestion that quality control criteria need to emerge from within a project rather than being applied from the outside. Quality control is more useful and coherent when it is tailored towards the project being undertaken and fits the topic and method. Reviewers need to select suitable quality evaluation benchmarks, justify their choices, and demonstrate how their projects meet these standards. The following three steps illustrate one way to implement a relativist viewpoint to systematic reviews:

- *Identify values or criteria underpinning the project*: Investigators can begin identifying their values when writing their review protocols.
- *Select methods that uphold those values and criteria*: Investigators then select methods that help them to uphold their values as they conduct their projects.
- *Present these values and methods to the reader*: Reviewers might, for example, include a table that links the methods to the values or criteria.

By identifying values and strategies when writing their protocols, reviewers are building quality control into their projects, rather than getting to the end and facing the task of having to show their work is of an adequate standard.

For example, researchers have explored how youth sport coaches interpret and make sense of their interactions with athletes, parents, colleagues, and administrators. Studies typically involve qualitative methods, and investigators have examined different types of coaches from various sports, locations, and environments. An aggregative review is unlikely to represent the findings with the same depth of insight as a configural synthesis, given the likely heterogeneity in the data. Further, an objective checklist may not be sufficiently tailored to evaluate the review beyond superficial criteria such as, was there a clear question? Did the authors detail their search? In drawing on a relativist approach, authors identify their values and underlying purposes for the study. These could be presented in their report as:

>> We aimed to (a) provide a clear answer to the question (b) evaluate primary studies from their own method perspective, (b) focus on understanding the humans who were the participants in the primary studies, (c) provide a story that advanced knowledge, (d) detail findings that other researchers and stakeholders would find engaging, (e) uncover our assumptions, (f) be transparent and methodical, (g) explore ethical considerations of our work, and (h) provide useful information for practitioners.

The authors could then provide a table in which they detail how they observed these values in concrete and behavioural terms. The text might read:

» To achieve these aims, we (a) wrote a protocol and had it reviewed by colleagues and stakeholders to ensure clarity of purpose and relevance for moving science forward, (b) identified suitable critical appraisal tools after finishing the search to ensure a match between primary study evaluation and method, (c) had a steering committee consisting of stakeholders, researchers, and coach educators to give us feedback on how engaging and practical the results were for them, and (d) invited the steering group to act as critical friends to help us reflect on our biases and the ethical considerations of the work.

One advantage for reviewers who identify their values and associated quality assurance behaviours is that they are communicating the suitable criteria by which to evaluate their work and are reducing the chance that readers will apply incompatible standards. Another advantage is that reviewers are being transparent with quality control. Readers might not agree with the benchmarks, but reviewers have the opportunity to explain and justify their decision-making.

Example Quality Criteria

Adopting a relativist viewpoint involves acknowledging the limitations of universal thinking and being open to moving among different criteria across reviews and even time within a project. From a non-foundational view, judging quality is both in the hands of the reviewer and the reader (Patton, 2015). To help reviewers consider and select criteria by which they can assess their work, the following list is an adaptation of the one Smith and Caddick (2012) proposed for qualitative research. Although Smith and Caddick suggest these benchmarks for qualitative research, it is useful to highlight the parallels between configural reviews and qualitative research: both involve subjective judgements and creative decision-making when synthesizing often ambiguous and heterogeneous information. There is seldom any objective reality against which to judge the results as true or false, and instead there is a focus on standards such as plausibility, coherence, and usefulness.

- *Substantive contribution*: Does the review contribute meaningfully to the understanding of social life?
- *Impact*: Does the review engage and influence the reader, perhaps stimulating a new perspective or new questions?
- *Width and depth*: Does the review provide sufficient evidence to support the knowledge and practice claims?
- *Coherence*: Does the review create a complete and meaningful story both in terms of how the sections fit together and connect with existing knowledge?
- *Change impetus*: Is the review likely to prompt action on the part of the reader?
- *Ethics*: Have the ethical implications of the review and its findings been considered?
- *Resonance*: Does the review affect or move the reader emotionally or behaviourally, as well intellectually?

- *Credibility*: Have the reviewers interacted with stakeholders sufficiently, perhaps inviting review and critique?
- *Transparency*: Is the review method transparent and justifiable?

The above principles are not presented as necessary or sufficient criteria for evaluating configural reviews. Instead, they are example yardsticks that might be present in a quality assessment toolbox from which reviewers can dip into when reflecting on the strength of their work. Similar to a carpenter's toolbox, reviewers can add or remove tools as befits their current work. Expertise in systematic reviewing involves knowing which tools are needed for which purposes, and being able to justify the selection. A relativist viewpoint allows reviewers the freedom to draw on their knowledge and interactions with stakeholders to ensure quality assessment is tailored to their needs.

Chapter Case Example: The Influence of Preoperative Exercise on People with Cancer

The case study for the current chapter focuses on the influence of preoperative physical exercise on postoperative complications, length of stay, and quality of life in patients with cancer (Steffens, Beckenkamp, Hancock, Solomon, & Young, 2018). The manuscript can be obtained from the *British Journal of Sports Medicine* and was published in 2018, Vol. 52, article number 344. In this chapter I examine the review through Liabo et al.'s (2017) lens.

Purpose   The purpose was to examine the effectiveness of preoperative exercise interventions (*PICO: Intervention*) in patients undergoing oncological surgery (*PICO: Population*), on postoperative complications, length of hospital stay, and quality of life (*PICO: Outcome*). The eligible control conditions included no intervention, placebo, or minimal intervention (*PICO: Comparison*).

Assessing the Review Method

Rigour   The review followed the Cochrane Collaboration guidelines and was written according to the PRISMA checklist. The authors developed a protocol according to the PRISMA-P format and registered it at PROSPERO. These behaviours help the reader to have confidence in the review's rigour, although making the PRISMA checklist publically available would have further enhanced credibility.

Suitability   The authors undertook a meta-analysis on controlled trials ensuring coherence between the question and the method. The review satisfied Liabo's et al. (2017) method suitability criteria.

Focus   In the report's introduction, the authors define postoperative complications, length of stay, and quality of life as three important variables associated with disease burden and distress following surgery. They reviewed controlled studies for these effects across any type of cancer. As such, the authors defend the review's coherent focus.

Assessing the Included Studies

Rigour   The authors used the Cochrane risk of bias tool, allowing for a rigorous assessment of the included trials. They found about 50% of the trials had at least one high risk of bias domain. These domains included risk of selection bias (allocation concealment), performance bias (blinding of participants and personnel) and detection bias (blinding of outcome assessment).

Design   The review limited the inclusion criteria to controlled trials. The inclusion criteria helped to ensure that the included studies were of a suitable design to allow a meaningful answer to the question.

Focus   Similarly, the reviewers designed the inclusion criteria to ensure that trials of exercise interventions, focused on people with cancer, and that measured the identified outcomes were included. These inclusion criteria helped to ensure that the primary research was of a suitable focus to allow meaningful answers.

10

Assessing the Evidence Synthesis

The authors concluded that across 13 trials, involving 806 participants and 6 types of cancer, there was moderate-quality evidence that preoperative exercise significantly reduced postoperative complication rates and length of hospital stay in patients undergoing lung resection. In patients with oesophageal cancer, preoperative exercise was not effective in reducing length of hospital stay. Further, although only assessed in single trials, preoperative exercise improved postoperative quality of life in patients with oral or prostate cancer. No effect was found in patients with colon and colorectal liver metastases.

The authors presented a GRADE summary of findings table. According to GRADE procedures, the quality of evidence across the outcomes for each cancer type varied from very low to low, except for lung cancer. In lung cancer, the evidence was of moderate quality for complications and hospital stay. These findings underscore the authors' conclusions that (a) preoperative exercise is effective in reducing postoperative complications and length of hospital stay in patients with lung cancer, and (b) the evidence is unclear if preoperative exercise reduces complications, reduces length of hospital stay, or improves quality of life in other groups of patients undergoing cancer surgery.

On the basis of the report, the review is of high quality and gives a rigorous up-to-date summary, as of 2018, of the influence of pre-surgery exercise on selected post-surgery variables. The review allows us to be confident that we do not know much.

Summary

Many reviews in sport, exercise, and physical activity include a paragraph on the project's strengths and weaknesses. Few authors, however, engage in a self-assessment as extensive as presented in this chapter. Nevertheless, critical self-reflection is helpful in establishing the confidence that we can have in the review's findings. When realizing that reviews, via professional practice and policy, influence people's lives then the critical appraisal of the project has real world implications beyond whether it is accepted or rejected for publication. Critical appraisal influences the interpretation of results and the conclusions authors present when disseminating their work, the topic of the next chapter.

❷ Learning Exercises

1. Select an aggregative review or meta-analysis on a topic that interests you. Visit the PRISMA and AMSTAR-2 websites and obtain their reporting standards checklists. Read the review and then critically appraisal it twice, once using the PRISMA tool and again with the AMSTAR-2 instrument. Compare the two tools:
   - Which seemed easier to use and had clearer instructions?
   - Did one helped you understand and evaluate the review more than the other?
   - Was there information missing from the tools that you thought needed to be added?
   - If a friend asked you for a recommendation, which tool would you suggest?
2. Obtain a configural review synthesizing qualitative research. Undertake the following exercise with a friend. Evaluate the review using the criteria presented above for configural reviews.
   - Start by each of you appraising the review independently of each other.
   - On completion, compare your assessments. Discuss and resolve variation and seek explanations for why you differed.
   - Together identify which of the criteria were relevant for the review and which seemed superfluous.
   - Together decide if there were additional criteria that may have been relevant.
3. Revisit the review you have been developing as you have been reading this book. In light of the current chapter:

   - Identify tools and criteria that you could use to ensure your review was of high quality.
   - Make a decision about how you will incorporate these tools and criteria into your project.
   - Update the protocol you wrote from ▶ Chapter 2.

References

Aronowitz, S. (1988). *Science as power: Discourse and ideology in modern society*. Minneapolis, MN: University of Minnesota Press.

Barnett-Page, E., & Thomas, J. (2009). Methods for the synthesis of qualitative research: A critical review. *BMC Medical Research Methodology, 9*, article 59. ▸ https://doi.org/10.1186/1471-2288-9-59.

Chalmers, I., & Altman, D. G. (1995). *Systematic reviews*. London, UK: BMJ Publishing.

Fanelli, D. (2012). Negative results are disappearing from most disciplines and countries. *Scientometrics, 90*, 891–904. ▸ https://doi.org/10.1007/s11192-011-0494-7.

Greenhalgh, T., Robert, G., Macfarlane, F., Bate, P., Kyriakidou, O., & Peacock, R. (2005). Storylines of research in diffusion of innovation: A meta-narrative approach to systematic review. *Social Science and Medicine, 61*, 417–430. ▸ https://doi.org/10.1016/j.socscimed.2004.12.001.

Guyatt, G., Oxman, A. D., Akl, E. A., Kunz, R., Vist, G., Brozek, J., … Schünemann, H. J. (2011). GRADE guidelines: 1. Introduction—GRADE evidence profiles and summary of findings tables. *Journal of Clinical Epidemiology, 64*, 383–394. ▸ https://doi.org/10.1016/j.jclinepi.2010.04.026.

Hammersley, M. (2006). Systematic or unsystematic, is that the question? Some reflections on the science, art, and politics of reviewing research evidence. In A. Killoran, C. Swann, & M. P. Kelly (Eds.), *Public health evidence: Tackling health inequalities* (pp. 239–250). Oxford, UK: Oxford University Press.

Ioannidis, J. P. A. (2005). Why most published research findings are false. *PLoS Medicine, 2*, article 124. ▸ https://doi.org/10.1371/journal.pmed.0020124.

Lewin, S., Glenton, C., Munthe-Kaas, H., Carlsen, B., Colvin, C. J., Gülmezoglu, M., … Rashidian, A. (2015). Using qualitative evidence in decision making for health and social interventions: An approach to assess confidence in findings from qualitative evidence syntheses (GRADE-CERQual). *PLoS Medicine, 13*, article 1001895. ▸ https://doi.org/10.1371/journal.pmed.1001895.

Liabo, K., Gough, D., & Harden, A. (2017). Developing justifiable evidence claims. In D. Gough, S. Oliver, & J. Thomas (Eds.), *An introduction to systematic reviews* (2nd ed., pp. 251–277). Thousand Oaks, CA: Sage.

Oliver, S. R., Rees, R. W., Clarke-Jones, L., Milne, R., Oakley, A. R., Gabbay, J., … Gyte, G. (2008). A multi-dimensional conceptual framework for analysing public involvement in health services research. *Health Expectations, 11*, 72–84. ▸ https://doi.org/10.1111/j.1369-7625.2007.00476.x.

Oreskes, N., & Conway, E. M. (2010). *Merchants of doubt: How a handful of scientists obscured the truth on issues from tobacco smoke to global warming*. New York, NY: Bloomsbury.

Patton, M. Q. (2015). *Qualitative research and evaluation methods* (4th ed.). Thousand Oaks, CA: Sage.

Pope, C., Mays, N., & Popay, J. (2007). *Synthesizing qualitative and quantitative health evidence: A guide to methods*. Maidenhead, UK: Open University Press.

Shah, I. (1966). *The exploits of the incomparable Mulla Nasrudin*. London, UK: ISF Publishing.

Shea, B. J., Reeves, B. C., Wells, G., Thuku, M., Hamel, C., Moran, J., … Henry, D. A. (2017). AMSTAR 2: A critical appraisal tool for systematic reviews that include randomised or non-randomised studies of healthcare interventions, or both. *British Medical Journal, 358*, article 4008. ▸ https://doi.org/10.1136/bmj.j4008.

Smith, B., & Caddick, N. (2012). Qualitative methods in sport: A concise overview for guiding social scientific sport research. *Asia Pacific Journal of Sport and Social Science, 1*, 60–73. ▸ https://doi.org/10.1080/21640599.2012.701373.

Sparkes, A. C., & Smith, B. (2014). *Qualiative research methods in sport, exercise, and health: From process to product*. Abingdon, OX: Routledge.

Steffens, D., Beckenkamp, P. R., Hancock, M., Solomon, M., & Young, J. (2018). Preoperative exercise halves the postoperative complication rate in patients with lung cancer: A systematic review of the effect of exercise on complications, length of stay and quality of life in patients with cancer. *British Journal of Sports Medicine, 52*, article 344. ▸ https://doi.org/10.1136/bjsports-2017-098032.

Tod, D., & Edwards, C. (2015). A meta-analysis of the drive for muscularity's relationships with exercise behaviour, disordered eating, supplement consumption, and exercise dependence. *International Review of Sport and Exercise Psychology, 8*, 185–203. ▸ https://doi.org/10.1080/1750984X.2015.1052089.

10

Disseminating Results

© The Author(s) 2019
D. Tod, *Conducting Systematic Reviews in Sport, Exercise, and Physical Activity*,
https://doi.org/10.1007/978-3-030-12263-8_11

Learning Objectives

After reading this chapter, you should be able to:
- Include elements needed for high quality reports.
- Work with stakeholders so that review findings influence targeted audiences.
- Engage in useful writing practices.
- Develop effective oral and poster presentations.

Introduction

» A scientific experiment, no matter how spectacular the results, is not completed until the results are published. In fact, the cornerstone of the philosophy of science is based on the fundamental assumption that original research must be published; only thus can new scientific knowledge be authenticated and then added to the existing database that we call scientific knowledge. (Gastel & Day, 2016, p. xv)

Research is a social activity and knowledge is a form of social capital. Investigators, readers, and communities only benefit from systematic reviews when they are publically disseminated. The majority of systematic reviews are communicated via the written word, and as Barrass's (2002) book title, *Scientists Must Write*, states clearly, writing is a necessary behaviour for researchers to survive in science.

In recent years, systematic reviews have proliferated rapidly. Page et al. (2016) estimated more than 8000 systematic reviews are being indexed in Medline per year, implying that greater than 22 are being published each day. Systematic reviews are not limited to medical and health topics, and the number being added to the scientific literature is likely much greater than 22 per day, any of which may be relevant to sport, exercise, and physical activity. Given the deluge of reviews, investigators need to consider how to make their work standout from the crowd and have an influence in the field. Learning ways to disseminate one's work helps investigators leave a legacy. In the current chapter I discuss ways to communicate systematic review findings, including elements needed in high quality reports, strategies for working with stakeholders, helpful writing practices, and components of effective oral and poster presentations.

Elements Needed for High Quality Reports

Over the past 30 years, a number of professional organizations have made concerted efforts to raise the quality of research reporting, particularly in medicine and health (Eden, Levit, Berg, & Morton, 2011). Two specific motivations for promoting standards in scientific publishing include ensuring influence and detecting biased reporting (Eden et al., 2011). Regarding influence, stakeholders, decision makers, and practitioners are more likely to consider the findings from well-presented research reports than from poorly written documents. With respect to biased reporting, investigators who produce clear, understandable, and complete publications will find it easier to demonstrate their work is rigorous, transparent, and credible, compared with individuals who write unclear, incomprehensible, and incomplete reports.

One consequence of these organizations' efforts has been numerous reporting standards or checklists encompassing items they deem required for adequate research documentation. For example, the Enhancing the QUAlity and Transparency of Health Research (EQUATOR) Network is a global enterprise seeking to improve the credibility and value of health research literature by advocating the use of robust reporting standards to ensure transparent and accurate documentation (▶ http://www. equator-network.org/about-us/). The EQUATOR website is a clearinghouse of standards for various types of research designs, a number of which will be familiar with sport, exercise, and physical activity investigators. For example, the website provides access to:

- The Consolidated Standards of Reporting Trials (CONSORT) checklist and flow diagram designed for randomized controlled trials (Moher et al., 2012).
- The Strengthening the Reporting of Observational Studies in Epidemiology (STROBE) Statement which details guidelines for reporting observational studies (von Elm et al., 2014).
- The Consolidated Health Economic Evaluation Reporting Standards (CHEERS) Statement for economic evaluations of health interventions (Husereau et al., 2013).
- The Standards for Reporting Qualitative Research (SRQR) for naturalistic investigations (O'Brien, Harris, Beckman, Reed, & Cook, 2014).

The arguments for reporting standards in primary research also apply to systematic reviews. The variation in the quality of primary research documentation is paralleled in systematic reviews (Pussegoda et al., 2017; Tricco et al., 2016; Zorzela et al., 2014). To illustrate, Page et al. (2016) surveyed 682 systematic reviews and found that a third or more failed to document (a) using a systematic review protocol, (b) eligibility criteria relating to publication status, (c) years of coverage of the search, (d) a full Boolean search for one or more databases, (e) data extraction methods, (f) critical appraisal methods, (g) a primary outcome, (h) an abstract conclusion that incorporated study limitations, or (i) the systematic review's funding source.

Incomplete or inconsistent reporting does not equate to a poorly conducted review (Eden et al., 2011). Investigators might have undertaken an excellent review of great quality, but failed to report their work adequately. Equally, a poorly implemented review may be presented in ways that make it appear a good piece of work. An incomplete report, however, lacks transparency and prevents readers from being able to make an informed judgement about the project's quality.

The inconsistent and poor reporting of systematic reviews has motivated scientific organizations to develop quality and reporting standards to help investigators conduct and disseminate projects that advance knowledge meaningfully and assist in effective decision-making. For example, the United States Committee on Standards for Systematic Reviews of Comparative Effectiveness Research developed three checklists of items that focused on: (a) the preparation of a final report, (b) the inclusion of peer review in report drafting, and (c) the publication of a report in a manner to allow open access (Eden et al., 2011). Currently, several other reporting standards exist. Examples on the EQUATOR website include:

- The Preferred Reporting Items for Systematic Reviews and Meta-Analyses (PRISMA) checklist and flow diagram tailored towards meta-analyses of randomized controlled trials (Moher, Liberati, Tetzlaff, Altman, & The Prisma Group, 2009).
- The Meta-analysis of Observational Studies in Epidemiology (MOOSE) guidelines for reviews of observational studies (Stroup et al., 2000).
- The RAMESES publication standards for meta-narrative reviews and realist syntheses (Wong, Greenhalgh, Westhorp, Buckingham, & Pawson, 2013a, 2013b).
- AMSTAR-2 (A Measurement Tool to Assess systematic Reviews) designed for systematic reviews that include randomised or nonrandomised studies of healthcare interventions (Shea et al., 2017).

Referring to publication guidelines prior to beginning, and during, a review assists investigators in designing and implementing excellent projects. They may then find it straightforward to write up high quality reviews, because all the necessary information is present and there are no gaps to address. Being in possession of a high quality review may mean that investigators are confident that stakeholders will value their work and it will generate impact or influence outside of academia.

Disseminating Systematic Reviews Among Stakeholders

Researchers, including some in sport, exercise, and physical activity, may believe their sole role is to generate new knowledge, and it is for others to use the results (Petticrew & Roberts, 2006). Their beliefs do not accord with the prevailing view among stakeholders and research consumers. Funders, such as the United Kingdom's research councils, for example, evaluate grant applications in part by investigators' plans for disseminating their work and ensuring their findings have an influence in society. The British government's periodic research assessment exercise, where investigators and research organizations have their work scrutinized for the purpose of allocating funding, includes criteria focused on impact. Researchers are required to demonstrate how their work has made a difference to people and communities.

Scientists' training at the postgraduate level generally includes little, if any, education on impact. In many sport, exercise, and physical activity-related university departments, impact education is typically limited to occasional workshops. Fortunately, other organizations provide resources to help researchers, such as the British research councils. To illustrate, the Economic and Social Research Council's (ESRC; ▶ https://esrc.ukri.org/) website contains information and resources that can help investigators in sport, exercise, and physical activity create impact among communities.

The ESRC describes impact as the contribution research makes to society and the economy, highlighting that it occurs when investigators and consumers interact, sharing their ideas, experiences, and skills. Science has influence when underpinned by collaboration; that is, when it is undertaken *with* rather than *on* people. Ways to promote collaboration include:

- Exploring the reasons why researchers and stakeholders want to work together and how they will benefit.

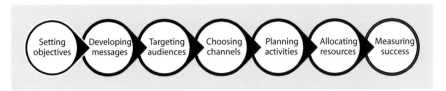

▣ **Fig. 11.1** The Economic and Social Research Council's steps in developing impact

- Deciding what the differrent groups bring to the project and what their responsibilities will include.
- Planning the logistics of the partnership and the daily activities.
- Discussing the financial, time, and other resources needed.
- Considering how to safeguard the project's sustainability and legacy.

Based on the projects the ESRC has funded, they have identified factors that help scientists promote positive impact, including:
- Establishing networks and relationships with stakeholders and research consumers.
- Acknowledging that stakeholders and research users have relevant knowledge and skills to help produce impact.
- Involving stakeholders and users at all stages of the research.
- Being flexible when working with partners and collaborators.
- Learning about the context and culture in which the research occurs.
- Committing to research activity that stakeholders want undertaken.
- Striving for excellent research infrastructure, leadership, and management.
- Recognizing that gatekeepers and brokers sometimes achieve more than investigators themselves.
- Engaging in collaborative reflection and assessment of the project and partnership.

A key component of building impact is the need for investigators to plan for and create influence rather than viewing it as a consequence that will happen without effort. The ESRC provides a step-by-step guide, illustrated in ▣ Fig. 11.1, that researchers can use, along with support materials (▶ https://esrc.ukri.org/research/impact-toolkit/developing-a-communications-and-impact-strategy/).

The seven steps in the ESRC's guide can be grouped into broader phases that are common to many goal setting and behaviour change models. The strategy begins with identifying the purpose and desired outputs of the strategy (step 1). For example, investigators undertaking a review of steroid prevention programmes might ask stakeholders what information they would find helpful and then use the responses to tailor the project's objectives.

The next phase involves the gathering of information which in this case involves identifying the key messages (that might change over the course of the partnership, step 2), the suitable audiences (step 3), and the effective communication channels (step 4). For the steroid prevention review, one key message might be that effective interventions are based on building good relationships with drug users. The suitable audiences could include staff working at needle exchange units, medical personnel, National Health Service management, and government officials. The effective communication channels would need to be tailored to each specific audience, but could involve workshops, placements, and websites, as well as traditional journal publications.

After gathering information, investigators plan the activities they will undertake (step 5), along with allocating the resources to allow those tasks to occur (step 6). The steroid prevention reviewers, for example, may work with stakeholders and targeted audiences to help arrange workshops, placements, websites, etc. Step seven includes measuring success. The steroid prevention investigators may, for example, collect data about how targeted audiences have reacted to their key messages, along with indicators of changes in policy, practices, or even drug use.

To help investigators implement the step-by-step guide effectively, the ESRC provides information and tools to assist with activities associated with communication and impact generation. These resources cover social media, websites, publications, educational materials, the media, events management, and policymakers. The ESRC provides the following tips to help researchers maximize the benefits from their communication and impact strategy:

- Begin your plan with clear, simple, and measurable objectives.
- Focus the impact and communication strategy goals on creating influence and avoid rewriting the project objectives.
- Write key messages in clear and accessible language.
- Pilot key messages to find the most effective ways of presenting them.
- Prioritize your target audiences according to their influence relative to your objectives.
- Tailor communication channels to the audience's preferences.
- When planning the strategy, include all the activities you intend to undertake, along with timelines, each partner's responsibilities, and costs.
- Avoid underestimating the resources needed to implement the plan.
- Prioritize high impact/low cost activities.
- Include the cost of hiring specialist help.
- Start measuring indicators of effectiveness before implementing the strategy.

Effective dissemination of review results may include workshops, websites, trade publications, or even more creative means, such as theatrical or musical productions. The effective vehicle is determined by factors external to the research group, such as the audience's preferences and available resources. The most frequent dissemination channel for systematic reviews in sport, exercise, and physical activity is the written word and scientific peer review journal publication. Writing well is a difficult craft to master, yet because it is necessary to the production of the majority of reviews in our domains, reviewers and postgraduate students benefit attending to the topic.

Habits of Effective Science Writers

Steven Covey's (1989) book, *The 7 Habits of Highly Effective People*, contains information that has helped many people organize their lives. The book's themes also have relevance for identifying helpful scientific writing practices.

Be Proactive

Steven Pinker (2015), cognitive neuropsychologist and popular science author, suggests that "writing is an unnatural act … and must be laboriously acquired" (p. 26). His argument applies to systematic reviews. People are not born knowing how to write systematic reviews (or other scientific documents). The challenge is to express and integrate complex ideas in the written form so that readers can understand them clearly and easily. Writing clear prose takes time and mental effort, and similar to other skills, such as playing the drum kit, needs to be learned. Anybody can hit drums, but that does not make her or him a musician. People need to learn several rudimentary movements and how to sequence them to produce a drum track that sounds pleasing to the ear. Sadly, no one is born a drummer and the same is true of writers. Like drumming, however, writing is a cognitive-motor skill that people can improve with coaching and practice.

Scientific writing is generally not an urgent task and people frequently find ways to avoid the activity. Most science writers in sport, exercise, and physical activity are people employed in roles involving many duties, such as teaching, researching, administration, and public service. There is always something to distract them. Writing occurs only when people deliberately structure their days to allow them time and space to engage in the task.

Begin with the End in Mind

A mental image of what their article, chapter, or book will look like may help science writers describe what they wish to achieve. Authors, for example, may write the abstract first, to clarify the content and order of their key messages. Another strategy is to obtain examples of what authors are hoping to produce, such as existing articles or manuscripts. Two conceptual features that assist people in developing a mental image include plot and style.

Plot   Plot refers to the sequencing of events and is as relevant for systematic reviews as for fiction. A common fiction plot starts with an exposition that introduces the main characters and setting. Tension is then built as the main characters undertake a series of tasks that result in the climax. The climax is the high point of the tension and is when authors offer solutions. Denouement comes after the climax when authors bring together and resolve the various plot strands. The fiction plot mirrors the structure of the typical systematic review. The introduction identifies the main conceptual characters, ideas, and contexts in a way to allows readers insights into the major task, which involves answering a review question. The method section builds tension by describing the tasks the researchers undertook to answer the question. The tension results from the reader's assessment of the method: is it valid, suitable, and relevant given the question? Authors need to meet readers' expectations for the review to be deemed high quality. The results section is the manuscript's climax because it answers the review's questions. Denouement occurs in the discussion where authors tie together the various strands from the results and position the review in the broader literature. Understanding plot helps authors give due emphasis to the various components. Paralleling fiction where everything needs to serve the story, in the systematic review, all components need to serve the answer to the question. For example, extended introductions and discussions containing irrelevant material are likely to distract readers from the review's knowledge contribution.

Style   Style refers to the way that authors express their ideas, and goes beyond the surface conventions regarding word and sentence arrangement, to include answers to questions about the author, the audience, their relationship with each other, and the goals of writing (deLaplante, 2016). There are various writing styles and they serve different purposes. For systematic reviews, two that are relevant include practical and reflective style (deLaplante, 2016).

Aggregative reviews, for example, often reflect a practical style in which writers focus on serving readers' needs. The reader has a gap in knowledge or a problem to solve. Reading is a means to an end, and not a goal in itself. The writer's primary objective is to maximize the efficiency at which readers can obtain the information from the document. In academic practical style, readers and writers share a collegial non-hierarchical relationship. Writers pitch their work at peers who wish to learn what the author knows. In practical style, the writing is ideally transparent, because the focus is on objective knowledge (deLaplante, 2016). The document is like a clean clear window through which readers can see the landscape or subject matter.

Configural reviews synthesizing qualitative research, however, may be based on a reflexive style in which authors draw readers' attention to the act of writing about a topic as well as to the subject matter. In reflexive writing, authors direct readers to the window as well as the landscape (deLaplante, 2016). The window is not clean or clear, but is dirtied or cracked by the author's biases and influences. Reflexive authors admit that the knowledge is not objective, but is influenced by the way they have presented the information. One example illustrating a reflexive style is hedging and qualifying, where authors strive to protect themselves from criticisms that the knowledge is inaccurate or unscientific. The extensive use of hedging and qualifying in academic writing illustrates that most scientific documents are not purely reflexive or practical.

Classic style   As a third option, Pinker (2015) argued that academics benefit from writing in the classic style. In classic style, the relationship between writer and author is viewed as a conversation in which prose provides a window to the world (Thomas & Turner, 2011). Writers attempt to present truths about the world in ways that allow readers to see what authors view. The classic writer views truth as clear, simple, and verifiable. The author strives to present the truth as the finished product and sufficient in itself to explain a phenomenon. No attention is given to the process of knowledge creation, or the writer's difficulty in mastering the truth (Pinker, 2015; Thomas & Turner, 2011).

Awareness of style helps authors make decisions about how to write. For example, to write in a classic style, authors will tend to (Pinker, 2015):

- Limit meta-discourse, where they acknowledge they are writing, such as signposting (e.g., telling readers what is to come or what has already been presented) and professional narcissism (e.g., where authors focus on themselves rather than the material).
- Curb unnecessary hedging and qualifying.
- Avoid clichés or structure them in new ways.
- Write about specific concrete details and eschew abstraction where possible.
- Favour active rather than passive language.

Pinker (2015) does not present his recommendations as laws that can never be broken. Authors have the discretion to decide what serves the messages they wish to share. Some signposting, for example, helps readers make sense of large amounts of complicated material, and qualifying claims can legitimately demonstrate the limits of knowledge.

Put First Things First

"First things first" is a phrase that speaks to self-management. One aspect of self-management includes structuring the environment to avoid distractions and promote the act of writing. For example, authors might switch off phones or kill wifi. Other authors may choose to write in rooms without windows and to close doors to prevent distractions. Systematic reviewers will likely benefit from making sure writing equipment, primary research, dictionaries, etc. are available to them when they work. Another aspect of self-management includes self-awareness, such as knowing when one works best and what motivates one to prioritize writing. Putting first things first also includes developing a plan for the work being written. A suitable plan could be developed by answering the journalistic questions of when, where, what, why, and how.

Think Win/Win

Scientific publishing is a win/win endeavour and not a win/loss game. Thinking win/win focuses on writing in ways that benefit both authors and readers. In science getting a manuscript accepted for publication is an author win. Publishing articles that are well cited and have impact is another win. Writers only win, however, when they help readers win. To assist readers, writers need to produce works that satisfy the knowledge and practical needs of research consumers. Ideally, the peer review process is structured so that failure to produce informative texts that help readers prevents authors from publishing.

Helping readers win includes both the content and the way it is presented. A strategy to ensure content is well presented is to follow any rules set by relevant scientific communities. When submitting to a journal, for example, authors abiding by the manuscript submission guidelines remove one reason their work might be rejected. Guidelines facilitate communication among colleagues. Deviations from guidelines may interfere with optimal communication. For example, poorly formatted manuscripts hinder peer reviewers from performing their task efficiently. Peer review is a voluntary role and in sport, exercise, and physical activity typically comes with limited rewards beyond intrinsic satisfaction and goodwill. Writers who do not follow the author guidelines closely are making life difficult for reviewers. Authors gain little benefit by making the reviewing task more troublesome than it is already.

With respect to content, authors increase their chances of having work accepted when they follow the plot discussed above and avoid the common mistakes that editors and reviewers frequently encounter. Common mistakes, among others, include the lack of a clear purpose statement, using introductions to review the literature, and failing to emphasise the work's contribution in the discussion. Articles lacking a clear consistent purpose are difficult to evaluate, because it is unknown what authors were attempting to achieve. Understandably, reviews and articles without clear purpose statements are at an increased risk of rejection.

Students get told to review the literature in a manuscript introduction, although such advice is incomplete and vague. Novice science writers may misinterpret the advice to mean they should produce a literature review. The introduction is not a literature review. The section is a place to introduce the central conceptual characters of the project, explain the purpose of the article, and justify the need for the study. Extended introductions can quickly cloud the reader's understanding of the topic.

Similarly, students get taught to relate their findings back to the literature in the discussion, although the advice is again nebulous and imperfect. A consequence of the advice includes lengthy discussions where novice writers repeat the findings they presented in the results and focus on the parallels between their work and existing research. Replication has a role in science, both in original research and systematic reviews, but discussions become descriptive and uncritical if authors limit themselves to highlighting parallels or differences. A major purpose of the discussion is to demonstrate how the findings have advanced knowledge, perhaps independently or in concert with previous work.

Seek First to Understand and Then to Be Understood

Pinker (2015) discusses the curse of knowledge which refers to our inability to put aside what we know and view a topic from the reader's standpoint. An example of the curse is when people who are lost ask for directions from a stranger and receive complicated replies. The directions are clear in the stranger's mind, but the lost individual is still befuddled. The musician Bruce Springsteen said that he writes songs with the audience in mind, and the science writers who adopt the same attitude may find their writing becomes clearer for readers, minimizing the effort needed for comprehension.

Related to the advice to consider the audience is the recognition that various social groups have different conventions of style. Adhering to those rules helps ease the reader's burden. There are, for example, numerous style guides, such as Strunk and White's (2014) *The Elements of Style* or Williams' (1990) *Style: Toward Clarity and Grace*. Social conventions vary across time and place (deLaplante, 2016), and there are no absolute authorities who dictate stylistic rules (apart from Ph.D. supervisors), but writers who conform to the standards of the community they wish to communicate with will find it easier to have their message received and accepted.

Synergize

Writing is an individual sport, but publishing is a team game. The productive science writer is similar to the professional golfer, because both spend lengthy amounts of time in solitude, practicing their craft. Like golfers, science writers also benefit from having a supportive team or network to help them develop their skill and assist them in profiting from their work. To develop their skill, writers get advice and feedback from various people including colleagues, writing coaches, editors, reviewers, and publishers. A similar set of people also help writers gain reward from their work by publishing and marketing manuscripts as books, journal articles, web pages, etc.

The supportive team also includes boosters. Scientific writing, like all genres, can be difficult, time consuming, and associated with self-doubt. The written word reveals the author to the reader's scrutiny. The prospect that a writer's work will be evaluated negatively can stimulate anxiety. Supportive encouraging individuals can reassure writers they are capable, will complete their work, and have something worth publishing. These supportive people do not need to offer advice, but just their belief can be enough.

Sharpen the Saw

Covey used the phrase "sharpen the saw" to describe the need to engage in self-maintenance, renewal, and improvement. For the science author, part of sharpening the saw is to seek ways to improve writing ability. Many ways exist to develop writing skill, but most of them can be summed up in Stephen King's (2000) recommendation to read and write a great deal. King's recommendation reflects research regarding deliberate practice (Ericsson & Pool, 2016): the more we write and focus on improving weaknesses, the better we get.

Reading serves many purposes for science writers. First, science writers attempt to present a picture of the world that reflects scientific understanding. Authors who immerse themselves in the literature will have more material to draw on than individuals who do not read. Science writers who read will produce documents that are more up-to-date, relevant, and substantial than those who do not study the literature. Second, reading engages authors in observational learning, and they become aware of the differences between effective and ineffective written communication. Third, reading outside one's discipline can help authors generate new ideas and ways to study, interpret, and present the material within their realm of expertise. For example, qualitative researchers and people undertaking configural reviews benefit from reading classic fiction, such as *Lord of the Files* (Golding, 1954), in which authors discuss fundamental themes of being human through their rich description of daily life.

Conference Oral Presentations and Posters

Conference oral presentations and posters are common vehicles by which systematic reviews are circulated among the sport, exercise, and physical activity communities. Whereas written documents, such as theses and publications, often have sufficient space to allow an in-depth description of the project, oral presentations and posters do not. Instead, oral presentations and posters are short stories, rather than novels, and serve different purposes to written documents. These forms of dissemination allow reviewers to communicate key messages, arouse the audience's interest in the findings, and network with interested stakeholders.

The challenge for systematic reviewers is to condense large, complicated, and highly technical projects to a 10 min presentation or an A0 size poster. The most common threats to good communication are probably the inclusion of too much detail, the curse of knowledge, and the lack of adequate preparation. Fortunately, Google and Google scholar searches yield a huge number of resources to help reviewers develop, produce, and deliver effective oral and poster presentations (e.g., Bourne, 2007; Erren & Bourne, 2007).

The threat that Google is unable to help with is the lack of adequate preparation. Allowing sufficient time to prepare influences the quality of a presentation. The preparation time can be used to learn about the audience and the event you are attending so you can tailor the presentation to fit the occasion. Individuals can also test their posters or presentations before the actual day to gain feedback about what works well and what can be improved. Also, you can seek out and assess examples to help you decide on the ingredients of excellent presentations. For example, TED talks (▶ https://www.ted.com/talks) can be a source of high quality presentations that will provide ideas. TED also publishes books that provide insights into giving good presentations.

11

Chapter Case Example: Prevalence of Eating Disorders in Dancers

In 2014, Arcelus, Witcomb, and Mitchell produced a high quality meta-analysis examining the prevalence of eating disorders in dancers, published in the *European Eating Disorders Review*, Vol. 22, pages 92–101. A pre-published version is available online at Loughborough University's online depository (▶ https://dspace.lboro.ac.uk/dspace-jspui/handle/2134/18993). Results revealed that the overall prevalence was 12.0% (16.4% for ballet dancers), 2.0% (4% for ballet dancers) for anorexia, 4.4% (2% for ballet dancers) for bulimia, and 9.5% (14.9% for ballet dancers) for eating disorders not otherwise specified. ◼ Table 11.1 presents an assessment of the article against the MOOSE reporting guidelines.

The review contained information for 24 of the 34 items which is above average for reviews in our field. Journal word count restrictions sometimes make it difficult to include every item of information listed in reporting guidelines. The *European Eating Disorders Review* journal limits review articles to 5000 words which forces authors to prioritize information. Further, it is often not mandatory to follow reporting guidelines unless required by journal editors, funders, or some other authority. The *European Eating Disorders Review* does ask that reviewers follow the PRISMA guidelines. The PRISMA guidelines are tailored towards meta-analyses of randomized controlled trials and may not be the best choice for reviews of other study designs, such as Arcelus et al. (2014).

Missing information does not always lessen a review's contribution. Arcelus et al. (2014), for example, did not present hypotheses (item 2), the qualifications of the people who undertook the search (item 7), or sources of funding (item 34). When information is missing, readers need to decide whether the absence is a fatal or nonfatal flaw.

Hypothesis, for example, is suitable when reviewers are testing theoretical propositions. In Arcelus et al., hypotheses were not needed because the authors were not testing theoretical propositions, but were estimating prevalence. Including hypotheses may not have added to the credibility of Arcelus et al. Sometimes, however, missing information does influence readers' assessments of the review. Frequently, for example, critical appraisal of primary research and grey literature searches are missing from systematic reviews published in the sport, exercise, and physical activity domains. A lack of critical appraisal prevents readers from learning about the quality of evidence underpinning review findings and a lack of a grey literature search may introduce publication bias to the results. Just as with primary research, there are few perfect systematic reviews. Rather than automatically disregarding a systematic review because it is missing some information, it is a better practice to evaluate the influence that the absent details might have had on the interpretation of the results and adjust one's estimation of the project's contribution accordingly. Arcelus et al. (2014) shows us that dancers are a high risk group for eating disorders, and their work makes a significant contribution to knowledge.

◼ **Table 11.1**   MOOSE checklist applied to Arcelus et al.'s (2014) meta-analysis

Reporting criteria	Yes/No	Page no.
Reporting of background		
Problem definition	Yes	92
Hypothesis statement	No	
Description of study outcome(s)	Yes	92–93
Type of exposure or intervention used	Yes	92–93
Type of study design used	Yes	93
Study population	Yes	92–93
Reporting of search strategy		
Qualifications of searchers	No	
Search strategy, including time period and keywords	Yes	93
Effort to include all available studies, including contact with authors	No	
Databases and registries searched	Yes	93
Search software used, name and version, including special features used (e.g., explosion)	Yes	93
Use of hand searching (e.g., reference lists of obtained articles)	Yes	93
List of citations located and those excluded, including justification	Yes	93–94
Method for addressing articles published in languages other than English	Yes	93
Method of handling abstracts and unpublished studies	Yes	93

(continued)

▣ Table 11.1 (continued)

Reporting criteria	Yes/No	Page no.
Description of any contact with authors	No	
Reporting of methods		
Description of relevance of studies assembled for assessing the hypothesis	Yes	93
Rationale for the selection and coding of data	Yes	93
Documentation of how data were classified and coded	Yes	93
Assessment of confounding	No	
Assessment of study quality	No	
Assessment of heterogeneity	Yes	93
Description of statistical methods in sufficient detail to be replicated	Yes	93
Provision of appropriate tables and graphics	Yes	95–99
Reporting of results		
Table giving descriptive information for each study included	Yes	95, 98–99
Results of sensitivity testing	Yes	94–95, 97
Indication of statistical uncertainty of findings	Yes	96
Reporting of discussion		
Quantitative assessment of bias	No	
Justification for exclusion	No	
Assessment of quality of included studies	No	
Reporting of conclusions		
Consideration of alternative explanations for observed results	Yes	97, 99–100
Generalization of the conclusions	Yes	99–100
Guidelines for future research	Yes	99–100
Disclosure of funding source	No	

11

Summary

» Writing is easy. All you do is stare at a blank sheet of paper until drops of blood form on your forehead. (Gene Fowler)

Regardless of the mechanism used to disseminate a systematic review, authors are going to use the written word in some way, either to express thoughts to others or to organize those thoughts beforehand. For scientists and reviewers, writing is a means to an end and not an end in itself. Good writing will assist reviewers in communicating their work so that their results contribute to knowledge, influences decision-making, and leaves a legacy. In the current chapter I have discussed ways that reviews can be communicated to achieve these end results. Effective communication is influenced by the quality of the review and in the penultimate chapter I focus on management topics that contribute to the completion of noteworthy projects.

❓ Learning Exercises

1. Locate a systematic review on a topic of your choice. After reading the report, visit the ESRC's (▶ https://esrc.ukri.org/) web pages dedicated to ensuring impact. Develop a plan for how you would ensure the review had an impact in the community. Specifically, identify the:
    — Key messages or implications contained in the review.
    — Audiences likely to benefit from these key messages or implications.
    — Stakeholder groups you could approach.
    — Resources that the stakeholders could provide.
    — Strategies by which to communicate the key messages to targeted audiences.
    — Changes you would hope to see.
    — Ways to evaluate the effectiveness of the communication strategies.
2. Locate a second systematic review on a topic that falls within an area with which you are familiar with. Read the review up until the end of the results section. Write a discussion that addresses the following topics:
    — A summary of the major findings.
    — The ways the findings advance knowledge in the area.
    — Applied implications that arise from the findings along with concrete suggestions about how they could be enacted to help specific groups of people.
    — The strengths and limitations of the review.
    — Possible avenues of future research that arise coherently from the results.
    — A clear conclusion that brings the review back to the topics contained in the review's opening paragraphs.
3. Using exercise one as a template, develop an impact strategy that could be relevant for the review you have been planning as you have been reading this book.

References

Arcelus, J., Witcomb, G. L., & Mitchell, A. (2014). Prevalence of eating disorders amongst dancers: A systemic review and meta-analysis. *European Eating Disorders Review, 22*, 92–101. ▶ https://doi.org/10.1002/erv.2271.

Barrass, R. (2002). *Scientists must write* (2nd ed.). London, UK: Routledge.

Bourne, P. E. (2007). Ten simple rules for making good oral presentations. *PLoS Computational Biology, 3*, article 77. ▶ https://doi.org/10.1371/journal.pcbi.0030077.

Covey, S. R. (1989). *The 7 habits of highly effective people*. New York, NY: Simon & Schuster.

deLaplante, K. (2016). The #1 misconception about writing style, from ▶ https://criticalthinkeracademy.com/courses/22120/lectures/315860.

Eden, J., Levit, L., Berg, A., & Morton, S. (2011). *Finding what works in health care: Standards for systematic reviews*. Washington, DC: National Academies Press.

Ericsson, A., & Pool, R. (2016). *Peak: Secrets from the new science of expertise*. London, UK: The Bodley Head.

Erren, T. C., & Bourne, P. E. (2007). Ten simple rules for a good poster presentation. *PLoS Computational Biology, 3*, article 102. ▶ https://doi.org/10.1371/journal.pcbi.0030102.

Gastel, B., & Day, R. A. (2016). *How to write and publish a scientific paper* (8th ed.). Cambridge, UK: Cambridge University Press.

Golding, W. (1954). *Lord of the flies*. London, UK: Faber and Faber.

Husereau, D., Drummond, M., Petrou, S., Carswell, C., Moher, D., Greenberg, D., … Loder, E. (2013). Consolidated health economic evaluation reporting standards (CHEERS) statement. *Cost Effectiveness and Resource Allocation, 11*, article 6. ▶ https://doi.org/10.1186/1478-7547-11-6.

King, S. (2000). *On writing: A memoir of the craft*. New York, NY: Scribner.

Moher, D., Hopewell, S., Schulz, K. F., Montori, V., Gøtzsche, P. C., Devereaux, P. J., … Altman, D. G. (2012). CONSORT 2010 explanation and elaboration: Updated guidelines for reporting parallel group randomised trials. *International Journal of Surgery, 10*, 28–55. ▶ https://doi.org/10.1016/j.ijsu.2011.10.001.

Moher, D., Liberati, A., Tetzlaff, J., Altman, D. G., & The Prisma Group. (2009). Preferred reporting items for systematic reviews and meta-analyses: The PRISMA statement. *PLoS Medicine, 6*, article 1000097. ▶ https://doi.org/10.1371/journal.pmed.1000097.

O'Brien, B. C., Harris, I. B., Beckman, T. J., Reed, D. A., & Cook, D. A. (2014). Standards for reporting qualitative research: A synthesis of recommendations. *Academic Medicine, 89*, 1245–1251. ▶ https://doi.org/10.1097/ACM.0000000000000388.

Page, M. J., Shamseer, L., Altman, D. G., Tetzlaff, J., Sampson, M., Tricco, A. C., … Moher, D. (2016). Epidemiology and reporting characteristics of systematic reviews of biomedical research: A cross-sectional study. *PLoS Medicine, 13*, article 1002028. ▶ https://doi.org/10.1371/journal.pmed.1002028.

Petticrew, M., & Roberts, H. (2006). *Systematic reviews in the social sciences: A practical guide*. Malden, MA: Blackwell.

Pinker, S. (2015). *The sense of style: The thinking person's guide to writing in the 21st century*. London, UK: Penguin Books.

Pussegoda, K., Turner, L., Garritty, C., Mayhew, A., Skidmore, B., Stevens, A., … Moher, D. (2017). Systematic review adherence to methodological or reporting quality. *Systematic Reviews, 6*, article 131. ▶ https://doi.org/10.1186/s13643-017-0527-2.

Shea, B. J., Reeves, B. C., Wells, G., Thuku, M., Hamel, C., Moran, J., … Henry, D. A. (2017). AMSTAR 2: A critical appraisal tool for systematic reviews that include randomised or non-randomised studies of healthcare interventions, or both. *British Medical Journal, 358*, article 4008. ▶ https://doi.org/10.1136/bmj.j4008.

Stroup, D. F., Berlin, J. A., Morton, S. C., Olkin, I., Williamson, G. D., Rennie, D., … Thacker, S. B. (2000). Meta-analysis of observational studies in epidemiology: A proposal for reporting. *Journal of the American Medical Association, 283*, 2008–2012. ▶ https://doi.org/10.1001/jama.283.15.2008.

Strunk, W., & White, E. B. (2014). *The elements of style* (4th ed.). Harlow, UK: Pearson.

Thomas, F. N., & Turner, M. (2011). *Clear and simple as the truth: Writing classic prose* (2nd ed.). Princeton, NJ: Princeton University Press.

Tricco, A. C., Lillie, E., Zarin, W., O'Brien, K., Colquhoun, H., Kastner, M., … Straus, S. E. (2016). A scoping review on the conduct and reporting of scoping reviews. *BMC Medical Research Methodology, 16*, article 15. ▶ https://doi.org/10.1186/s12874-016-0116-4.

von Elm, E., Altman, D. G., Egger, M., Pocock, S. J., Gøtzsche, P. C., & Vandenbroucke, J. P. (2014). The strengthening the reporting of observational studies in epidemiology (STROBE) statement: Guidelines for reporting observational studies. *International Journal of Surgery, 12*, 1495–1499. ▶ https://doi.org/10.1016/j.ijsu.2014.07.013.

Williams, J. M. (1990). *Style: Toward clarity and grace*. Chicago, IL: University of Chicago.

Wong, G., Greenhalgh, T., Westhorp, G., Buckingham, J., & Pawson, R. (2013a). RAMESES publication standards: Meta-narrative reviews. *BMC Medicine, 11*, article 20. ▶ https://doi.org/10.1186/1741-7015-11-20.

Wong, G., Greenhalgh, T., Westhorp, G., Buckingham, J., & Pawson, R. (2013b). RAMESES publication standards: Realist syntheses. *BMC Medicine, 11*, article 21. ▶ https://doi.org/10.1186/1741-7015-11-21.

Zorzela, L., Golder, S., Liu, Y., Pilkington, K., Hartling, L., Joffe, A., … Vohra, S. (2014). Quality of reporting in systematic reviews of adverse events: Systematic review. *British Medical Journal, 348*, article 7668. ▶ https://doi.org/10.1136/bmj.f7668.

11

Topics Related to Managing a Review

© The Author(s) 2019
D. Tod, *Conducting Systematic Reviews in Sport, Exercise, and Physical Activity*,
https://doi.org/10.1007/978-3-030-12263-8_12

Learning Outcomes

After reading this chapter, you should be able to:
- Discuss ethical considerations involved in systematic reviews.
- Evaluate software and technology that may assist a review.
- Decide when a review needs archiving, updating, or maintaining.

Introduction

In most domains of expertise, including sport, music, business, and science, technical knowledge and skills are necessary but insufficient for high productivity. In addition, having contextual knowledge and being able to predict, avoid, or navigate obstacles helps experts realize desirable outcomes. A similar principle applies in systematic reviews. Understanding how to run a meta-analysis, synthesis qualitative evidence, or search the grey literature are examples of technical skills. Knowing how to apply those skills given particular circumstances contributes to investigators producing influential reviews that are relevant, timely, meaningful, and ethically sound. Examples of additional useful knowledge and skills I address in the penultimate chapter include knowing how to act in ethical ways, how to make the best use of information management tools, and when to archive, update, and maintain a review.

Ethical Considerations

Academic Misconduct

12

In 2015, the *Indian Journal of Dermatology* retracted the article "Development of a guideline to approach plagiarism in Indian scenario" … for plagiarism (Anonymous, 2015). In a potentially more serious example of misconduct in science, New Zealand medical investigators reviewed 33 randomized controlled trials from one research group and concluded there were "inconsistencies between and within trials, errors in reported data, misleading text, duplicated data and text, and uncertainties about ethical oversight" (Bolland, Avenell, Gamble, & Grey, 2016, p. 2391). Subsequently, 21 of the 33 trials have been retracted (University of Auckland, 2018). Potentially, scientific misconduct has serious consequences that may include loss of life when patients are given ineffective or harmful treatments. Investigators in the sport, exercise, and physical activity fields examine aspects of physical, psychological, and social well-being, and the consequences of misconduct in our disciplines may also influence people's health.

Scientific misconduct refers to fabrication, falsification, and plagiarism (Gross, 2016). Gross (2016) states further that fabrication involves making up data or results. Falsification involves manipulating research materials, equipment, processes, data, or results. Plagiarism is the appropriation of another person's ideas, processes, results, or words without giving them credit. In addition to misconduct, scientists may engage in other unacceptable practices such as embezzlement of grant money, rounding *p*-values in desired directions, bullying, and ghost writing (where people with conflicts of interest write an article that when published is credited to another individual).

Studying scientific misconduct shares parallels with investigating doping in elite sport, because both behaviours occur in competitive environments and are not socially approved actions. Regarding prevalence, there are indications that scientific misconduct is not isolated to a few rotten apples in the scientific barrel. Approximately 2% of scientists admit to having engaged in plagiarism, falsification, or fabrication, with about 30% indicating they have observed colleagues undertaking such behaviours (Fanelli, 2009; Pupovac & Fanelli, 2015). If a broader range of questionable actions are included, such as deliberately not reporting unfavourable results, rounding *p*-values, or selectively reporting studies, then the rates are considerably higher (e.g., >75%, John, Loewenstein, & Prelec, 2012). As with doping in elite sport, there is always the suspicion that these rates underestimate prevalence.

Regarding motivation, scientific misconduct is associated with results-oriented cultures underpinned by the publish or perish ethos (Fanelli, Costas, Fang, Casadevall, & Bik, 2019). Further, misconduct occurs where robust social control and clear national policies are absent, and when productivity is linked with financial and other incentives (Fanelli et al., 2019). The parallels with elite sport are obvious for individuals who have worked in both environments.

Scientific organizations treat academic misconduct seriously. In addition to threatening the welfare of individuals and communities, misconduct damages the productivity and reputations of scientists, their institutions, and their colleagues (Azoulay, Bonatti, & Krieger, 2017; Hussinger & Pellens, 2019). Most people producing systematic reviews typically operate in the same environments as other researchers and may also be tempted to engage in academic misconduct or other questionable behaviours. The combination of protocol registration and adherence to reporting standards may help to reduce misconduct in systematic reviews, because they encourage transparency and full disclosure of relevant information. Most funders, universities, and other research-oriented organizations have codes of practice and other resources that reviewers can access to become familiar with stakeholder expectations and misconduct procedures. For example, the United Kingdom Research Integrity Office (UKRIO, n.d.) has a checklist to help investigators engage in good practice before, during, and after their projects (▶ http://ukrio.org/).

Ethics in Publishing

Related to scientific misconduct is ethics in publishing. Systematic reviewers may avoid difficulties and potential pitfalls by becoming aware of the typical ethical expectations when they disseminate their work in published form. Various organizations can help.

The Committee On Publishing Ethics (COPE) is one example. COPE assists scholarly journal editors, publishers, and other groups (e.g., funders) in promoting and maintaining publication integrity. The committee provides guidance on policies and practices to reflect transparency and integrity. The COPE websites contain a range of resources including flowcharts, webinars, and online courses. Their 10 core practices address:

- Allegations of misconduct.
- Authorship and contributorship.
- Complaints and appeals.
- Conflicts of interest.
- Data and reproducibility.
- Ethical oversight.
- Intellectual property.
- Journal management.
- Peer review processes.
- Post-publication discussions and corrections.

Most publishers of scientific material are members of COPE, and they also have their own policies and procedures. Palgrave Macmillan, for example, presents their policies and procedures online (▶ https://www.palgrave.com/gb/journal-authors/ethics-policy/10052358) and detail the responsibilities of authors, editors, reviewers, and the publisher. According to the Palgrave website, for example, authors should:

- Only submitted original and fully referenced research.
- Accurately present authors.
- Declare that their submissions are not being reviewed elsewhere.
- Provide accurate contact details for the corresponding author.
- Disclose sources of data and third party material.
- Identify third party material and obtain copyright permission.
- Disclose conflicts of interest.
- Agree to publication terms.
- Expect editors to scan submissions for plagiarism.
- Comply with editor or publisher requests for source data, proof of authorship, or evidence of originality.
- If unable to comply, provide reasonable explanations.
- Co-operate with any editor or publisher investigations.
- Expect transparency, efficiency, and respect from the publisher and editor.
- Communicate in good faith with the publisher and editor.
- Submit corrigenda, if needed, in a timely and responsible fashion.
- If needed, co-operate with the publication of errata or article retraction.

These guidelines may appear overwhelming. Authors, however, who make genuine attempts to behave in honest and transparent ways, and who respect the rights of others, are unlikely to willingly violate ethical principles or engage in misconduct.

Software and Information Technology Tools

The amount of information generated in a review can be tremendous and access to information technology can be useful. Tod and Edwards' (2015) meta-analysis on the relationships between the drive for muscularity and health-related behaviours illustrates the amount of data that can be recorded in a modest review. ◻ Figure 12.1 presents an estimate of information. As detailed in ◻ Fig. 12.1, at each stage of the review the number of active studies still left in the project decreased, but the amount of data

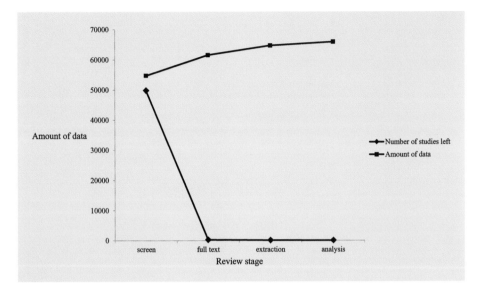

□ Fig. 12.1   Amount of data at each stage of Tod and Edward's (2015) review

available to the researchers to complete and write up the review increased. During the write up stage, although only 77 studies were left active, approximately 65,000 bits of information were available. Much of the information was focused on reasons why studies had been excluded and was captured during the search. Nevertheless, approximately 3500 bits of information were directly related to the analysis of the final 77 studies. Larger projects will extract more information than Tod and Edwards' review, and having access to information technology will assist in managing that level of knowledge.

   □ Table 12.1 details the various stages in which information management tools can help a reviewer. The table is based on the search engine at the systematic review toolbox web site (▶ http://systematicreviewtools.com/index.php). There are multiple tools at each stage and the table presents just one example. Some tools are open source and free, whereas others are commercial products. Some tools assist with multiple tasks in a review, and others focus on one activity. Some tools assist with several types of review, whereas others assist with just one kind of synthesis. For example, metaXL assists people completing a meta-analysis. Software such as NVivo may be helpful for configural reviews of qualitative research. Individuals who conduct multiple projects may benefit from exploring the systematic review toolbox's search engine.

   Brunton, Graziosi, and Thomas (2017) present reasons why information technology helps reviewers. First, software helps individuals make their reviews transparent and replicable through the recording and management of information. Second, software can prevent the loss or distortion of information. Third, effective management of data assists reviewers in defending decisions by allowing access to information, such as the reasons why specific investigations were excluded. Fourth, software can assist with archiving information, allowing reviewers the opportunity to update or amend their projects, the focus of the next section.

◻ **Table 12.1**   Stages in a systematic review for which systematic review toolbox lists possible information technology software

Review feature	Example
Protocol develop-ment	Systematic Review Accelerator (weblink: ► http://crebp-sra.com/#/)
Automated search	Article-based PubMed Search Engine (APSE) (weblink: ► https://pubmed.ict.griffith.edu.au/)
Study selection	Abstrackr (weblink: ► http://abstrackr.cebm.brown.edu/account/login)
Quality assessment	Covidence (weblink: ► https://www.covidence.org/home)
Data extraction	DistillerSR (weblink: ► https://www.evidencepartners.com/)
Automated analysis	Doctorevidence (weblink: ► http://drevidence.com/products/doc-data/)
Text analysis	Carrot2 (weblink: ► http://project.carrot2.org/)
Meta-analysis	MetaXL (weblink: ► http://www.epigear.com/index_files/metaxl.html)
Report write-up	Web-Based AMSTAR checklist (weblink: ► http://amstar.ca/Amstar_Checklist.php)
Collaboration	Cadima (weblink: ► https://www.cadima.info/index.php/area/evidenceSynthesisDatabase)
Reference manage-ment	Publish or Perish (weblink: ► https://harzing.com/resources/publish-or-perish)

12 Archiving, Updating, and Maintaining Reviews

Archiving Reviews

In many countries, storage and availability of primary data and personal information is a feature of research governed by various laws, ethical principles, and organizational policies. Such governance may be less applicable to systematic reviews, because data is often extracted from publically available sources (e.g., research publications). Also, the review's data may be presented in evidence tables contained within reports, or in the case of journal publication, supplementary files archived online. Although the various laws and regulations have been developed with a focus on primary research, they are models of good practice that systematic reviewers may choose to observe (Centre for Reviews and Dissemination, 2009). It would also be prudent for reviewers to establish with funders, publishers, and other relevant stakeholders any expectations about topics such as storage, access, and intellectual property (Rees & Oliver, 2017).

Decisions about what information to archive may also be influenced by the investigators' plans to maintain or update their projects. Even if reviewers, however, do not intend on updating a review, it may be sensible to archive as much information as possible so that if their ambitions change, or if new individuals develop the desire, then the data is available. The Centre for Reviews and Dissemination (2009) suggest the following information is retained, both electronically and physically:

- Extracted data.
- Critical appraisal data.
- Decisions made during the literature search, screening, extraction, and analysis.
- Meeting minutes.
- Correspondence and formal interactions with stakeholders and external parties.
- Feedback from peers and reviewers.
- The final report and earlier drafts.
- The original primary research, especially those documents difficult to reproduce such as conference abstracts, grey literature, and personal communications with authors.
- Copies of webpages and their uniform resource locators (URL).

The reason for keeping paper copies of information is because electronic files may become obsolete, lost, or corrupted.

As the move towards open science gathers momentum, the expectation that systematic review data and other information is publically available and free will become more widespread than it is currently. Organizations such as the Cochrane Collaboration, the Campbell Collaboration, the Joanna Briggs Institute, universities, and government departments already operate repositories that make reviews, data, and other materials freely available online. As a further example, the Systematic Review Data Repository (▶ https://srdr.ahrq.gov/) is an online archive of healthcare-related systematic review data. The creators at Brown University aim to maintain a clearinghouse of systematic review data which may be critiqued, updated, and augmented on an ongoing basis. The belief is that the database will facilitate evidence reviews and improve policymaking in healthcare.

What Is Updating?

Systematic reviewers aim to provide a synthesis of knowledge that is up-to-date and based on, typically, all the available evidence. Science is expanding, however, and some topics have a short half-life, defined as the length of time it takes for half the knowledge in an area to be disproved or become obsolete (Arbesman, 2013). To stay relevant, systematic reviews need to be updated on a regular basis.

Definitions of updating vary (Elkins, 2018), but it is useful to consider the Cochrane Collaboration's explanation, because of the organization's influence on systematic reviews in sport, exercise, and physical activity domains. The Cochrane Collaboration differentiates between *updates* and *amendments* (Higgins, Green, & Scholten, 2011), with a key difference being the inclusion of a search. Updates are defined as "any modification to the published document that includes the findings (including that of no new studies) from a more recent search for additional included studies than the previous published review" (p. 3.5). Amendments are "any modification or edit (including withdrawal) that does not include an update" (p. 3.6). The definitions highlight that updating a review is not limited to the inclusion of studies appearing after the publication of the original synthesis.

Beyond the inclusion of new evidence, there are several ways that individuals may update or amend reviews (Elkins, 2018; Higgins et al., 2011). Researchers, for example, are continuously developing new data collection methods, creating innovative analysis techniques, discovering novel outcomes, identifying fresh correlates, repackaging tired interventions, or proposing original theories. Investigators might update a review by analysing existing data with new statistical methods or interpreting qualitative studies through a novel theoretical lens. As long as reviewers had untaken a new search (and even if they had found no new studies), the Cochrane Collaboration would consider the outcome as an update.

How Often Should Reviewers Update Their Projects?

There are few studies or guidelines to inform investigators on how often to update their reviews (Garritty, Tsertsvadze, Tricco, Sampson, & Moher, 2010). Some groups have proposed strategies for determining whether a review needs to be updated, but the methods lack evidence (Elkins, 2018; Moher et al., 2008). The Cochrane Collaboration suggests reviews should be updated every two years (Higgins et al., 2011), but also acknowledges that some will need to be revised either more or less frequently, because knowledge advancement proceeds at various rates across topic areas. The limited evidence suggests that some reviews may not need updating for several years (>5.5), others will need revision within a year, and a few will be out of date by the time they are available (Shojania et al., 2007).

To decide if a review deserves to be updated or amended, investigators need to determine whether the result will (a) advance, extend, or challenge current knowledge, or (b) provide a firmer basis for decision-making. At a minimum, a preliminary search of the topic area will help investigators make their decision. To further assist reviewers, ▣ Table 12.2 presents a three step set of questions that emerged from a recent workshop on the topic (Garner et al., 2016). Change is a key theme running through the questions. If there are no new studies or alternative ways to synthesize the existing database, then it is unlikely that the review needs updating, especially if the original project was of high quality.

More specific questions that reviewers can ask when considering if their topic needs updating include (Elkins, 2018; Higgins et al., 2011):

— Are the objectives still relevant or do they need changing?
— Are there additional studies available to broaden, deepen, or provide alternative answers to the question?
— Will splitting the review into two or more projects advance knowledge better than keeping it as one investigation?
— Will the project benefit from retaining the existing authors or changing the people involved?

⬛ **Table 12.2** Garner et al.'s (2016) three step set of questions for updating a review
Step 1: Assess the review's currency Does the review address a current relevant question? Has the review had good access or use? Did the review employ valid methods and was it well conducted?
Step 2: Identify relevant new methods, studies, and other information Do new relevant methods exist? Are there new studies or other relevant types of evidence?
Step 3: Assess the effect of updating the review Will the new methods change the findings or credibility? Will the new studies, information, or data change the findings or credibility?

— In what ways has the world changed that justifies updating the project?
— In what ways can feedback from peers and other stakeholders inform a decision to update the review?
— Will the review help to clarify our understanding of the topic area?

In some areas of science, multiple reviews on the same or similar topics are appearing in the literature, sometimes with conflicting results (Ioannidis, 2016). The presence of multiple reviews with contradictory results hinders understanding of a topic. New reviews are wasteful unless they can reconcile differences or add a new understanding to the topic. For example, since 1997, there have been over 300 published papers focused on muscle dysmorphia (a diagnosable psychological disorder involving an obsession with building a muscular physique and compulsive behaviours such as weight training, disordered eating, and steroid abuse). Among that literature, there have been over 200 scientific investigations and approximately 70 reviews. There have been almost 10 systematic reviews or meta-analyses, and they reach the same conclusion: we do not know much about the condition because the majority of the research has been of poor quality. Until reviewers adopt a different perspective on the topic or the amount of high quality research published is increased considerably, then additional systematic reviews are unlikely to make meaningful increments to knowledge. They will advance people's careers, but not science.

Maintaining Reviews

The expansion of the science industry and the increasing rate of publication (Bastian, Glasziou, & Chalmers, 2010) shortens the time a review is up-to-date with the evidence base. People have searched for solutions to allow reviews to stay current, such as the Systematic Review Data Repository described above. Another response is the *living systematic review*, defined as a project "that is continually updated, incorporating relevant new evidence as it becomes available" (Elliott et al., 2017, p. 24). A central challenge in living reviews (or any other type) is the frequency of literature surveillance. There needs to be a balance between currency and feasibility because continual searching and updating takes time and resources. Elliott et al. recently suggested living systematic reviews are suitable when:

- They are necessary for making practice-based decisions and policy.
- There exists low levels of certainty in current knowledge.
- The research field is fast moving and new studies are being continuously published.

Traditional scientific publication channels are often not swift enough to allow living reviews to occur because of factors such as article publication lag time. Recent innovations, however, show promise in helping to speed up all tasks in a literature synthesis enabling the birth of living systematic reviews. Examples include machine learning, computer automation, standardization of activities, involvement of citizen scientists, crowdsourcing, and advances in meta-analysis techniques (Simmonds, Salanti, McKenzie, & Elliott, 2017; Thomas et al., 2017).

Recently, Elliot et al. (2017) provide guidance on how to develop and undertake living systematic reviews:

- Keep end users in mind.
- Minimize the workload for authors, peer reviewers, editors, and publishers.
- Maximize the visibility of the latest findings for readers.
- Maximize efficiencies through technology and crowdsourcing.
- Streamline workflow and editorial procedures.
- Build on, rather than reinventing, existing procedures and platforms.
- Focus on workable, not perfect, solutions.
- Remain flexible to incorporate new developments in the broader evidence ecosystem.

Elliot et al.'s principles reflect useful advice for all projects synthesizing research, not only living systematic reviews.

12

Chapter Case Example: Does Physical Fitness Training Benefit Stroke Patients?

The current chapter's case example focuses on the influence that fitness training has on stroke patients. The review is one that has been updated on multiple occasions and has had its conclusions changed several times. The original report appeared in the Cochrane Collaboration database in 2004 (Saunders, Greig, Young, & Mead, 2004). The most recent version appeared in 2016 (Saunders et al., 2016). The reports are open access and freely available from the Cochrane Database of Systematic Reviews.

Review purpose

The primary purpose was to assess if fitness training after stroke influences death, dependence, and disability. The secondary purpose was to evaluate the effects of training on adverse events, risk factors, physical fitness, mobility, physical function, quality of life, mood, and cognitive function. The original review in 2004 did not examine cognitive function, but the investigators included this class of outcomes in 2016 because it had been identified as a highly rated priority and had received research attention.

History of changes

Pages 408–409 of the 2016 report presents two tables, labelled "What's New" and "History," detailing the various changes the project has undergone since 2004. These changes include (Saunders et al., 2016):

- 2008, October: Reformatting the review.
- 2008, November: New search that realised 12 additional trials that were incorporated into the review and resulted in a new version of the project with modified conclusions.
- 2009, March: New search performed.
- 2010, November: New search that yielded 18 additional investigations that were incorporated into the review. There was a revision of authorship, inclusion criteria, objectives, main text, and conclusions.
- 2013, January: New search performed yielding 13 additional studies. The authors incorporated new risk of bias tables.
- 2013, July: The authors added a new author and revised main text and conclusions.
- 2015, October: A new search added 13 studies (the database now has 58 trials). Cognitive function added as an outcome, two new authors included, and conclusions revised.
- 2015, November: The review was recognised as a new version.

Change in conclusions

Based on 12 trials involving 289 participants, Saunders et al. (2004) concluded there was insufficient data to inform clinical practice. More generally, further trials were needed to examine the efficacy, feasibility, content, and type of physical training on stroke, especially soon after the event.

In the 2016 version of the review, Saunders et al. (2016) concluded there was sufficient evidence to include cardiorespiratory and mixed training, involving walking, into usual stroke care to reduce disability. Also training could be introduced subsequent to usual post-stroke care to enhance walking speed, tolerance, and perhaps balance. There was also sufficient evidence to include resistance training. Cardiorespiratory and mixed training (to a lesser extent) reduced disability. The effects of training on death and dependence were unclear, but these events rarely occurred in trials. Finally, further research was needed to examine cognitive function, long terms outcomes, and dose-response relationships.

The conclusions have changed a great deal in 12 years. One explanation for why the conclusions may have changed over time is that the review methods or the reviewers' perspectives had altered. In the current example, however, the reviewers have provided a history of their project, documented alterations, and made their reports publically available. These steps allow readers to compare the original and altered versions of the review and be in a position to decide if the differing conclusions reflect the accumulating evidence or rival explanations. In the current example, the updated conclusions appear to reflect the increased evidence.

Summary

In the words of jazz musicians, Sy Oliver and James Young:

» *'Tain't what you do; it's the way that you do it,*
'Tain't what you do; it's the time that you do it
That's what gets results

Their words have relevance for systematic reviewers. Teams that have the requisite technical knowledge, skills, and competencies to synthesis literature systematically to a high level of quality will produce fine documents. Technical aptness combined with contextual knowledge contributes to those same teams producing, maintaining, and updating relevant, influential, and ethical reviews over a number of years. Returning to Oliver and Young:

» *You've learned your A B C's,*
You've learned your D F G's,
But this is something you don't learn in school

In the final chapter I present the words of expert methodologists and reviewers. I asked them to give me their top advice for conducting reviews. Not all their suggestions appear in systematic review textbooks, but they do help shed light on how to undertake a project.

? Learning Exercises

12

1. Locate and read a systematic review that is more than five years old. Using the strategy described in the paper, undertake a search using one or two electronic databases, such as Google Scholar or PubMed, and order the results chronologically. Use Garner et al.'s 3 step procedures (presented in ◘ Table 12.2) to decide if the review needs updating. If so, respond to the following questions:
   - Is there a need to change the question? Why or why not?
   - Based on your preliminary search, how many studies have you identified might be added?
   - Is there a need to split the existing review into multiple projects?
   - Are there alternative methods that may help to answer the question?
2. Elliot et al. (2017) provided guidance on how to structure a protocol for a living systematic review. The article is available in the *Journal of Clinical Epidemiology*, Vol. 91, pages 23–30 (► https://www.jclinepi.com/article/S0895-4356(17)30636-4/fulltext). An author version is also available at researchgate. Obtain a copy and read the paper, noting Box 3 and Section 5. Then turning to the protocol you have developed as you have read this book:
   - Decide if your selected area is suitable for a Living Systematic Review.
   - Regardless of your answer to the above, make adjustments to your protocol so that it reflects an attempt to develop a Living Systematic Review.

3. Obtain a copy of UKRIO's checklist of good practice (▶ http://ukrio.org/ wp-content/uploads/UKRIO-Recommended-Checklist-for-Researchers.pdf). Use it to evaluate the ways in which your protocol needs adapting to ensure you will adhere to the UKRIO's guidance.

References

Anonymous. (2015). Development of a guideline to approach plagiarism in Indian scenario: Retraction. *Indian Journal of Dermatology, 60*, 210. ▶ https://doi.org/10.4103/0019-5154.152545.

Arbesman, S. (2013). *The half-life of facts: Why everything we know has an expiration date*. London, UK: Penguin.

Azoulay, P., Bonatti, A., & Krieger, J. L. (2017). The career effects of scandal: Evidence from scientific retractions. *Research Policy, 46*, 1552–1569. ▶ https://doi.org/10.1016/j.respol.2017.07.003.

Bastian, H., Glasziou, P., & Chalmers, I. (2010). Seventy-five trials and eleven systematic reviews a day: How will we ever keep up? *PLoS Medicine, 7*, article 1000326. ▶ https://doi.org/10.1371/journal. pmed.1000326.

Bolland, M. J., Avenell, A., Gamble, G. D., & Grey, A. (2016). Systematic review and statistical analysis of the integrity of 33 randomized controlled trials. *Neurology, 87*, 2391–2402. ▶ https://doi. org/10.1212/WNL.0000000000003387.

Brunton, J., Graziosi, S., & Thomas, J. (2017). Tools and technologies for information management. In D. Gough, S. Oliver, & J. Thomas (Eds.), *An introduction to systematic reviews* (2nd ed., pp. 145–180). Thousand Oaks, CA: Sage.

Centre for Reviews and Dissemination. (2009). *Systematic reviews: CRD's guidance for undertaking reviews in health care*. York, UK: Author.

Elkins, M. R. (2018). Updating systematic reviews. *Journal of Physiotherapy, 64*, 1–3. ▶ https://doi. org/10.1016/j.jphys.2017.11.009.

Elliott, J. H., Synnot, A., Turner, T., Simmonds, M., Akl, E. A., McDonald, S., … Thomas, J. (2017). Living systematic review: 1. Introduction—The why, what, when, and how. *Journal of Clinical Epidemiology, 91*, 23–30. ▶ https://doi.org/10.1016/j.jclinepi.2017.08.010.

Fanelli, D. (2009). How many scientists fabricate and falsify research? A systematic review and meta-analysis of survey data. *PloS One, 4*, article 5738. ▶ https://doi.org/10.1371/journal.pone.0005738.

Fanelli, D., Costas, R., Fang, F. C., Casadevall, A., & Bik, E. M. (2019). Testing hypotheses on risk factors for scientific misconduct via matched-control analysis of papers containing problematic image duplications. *Science and Engineering Ethics, 25*, 771–789. ▶ https://doi.org/10.1007/s11948-018-0023-7.

Garner, P., Hopewell, S., Chandler, J., MacLehose, H., Akl, E. A., Beyene, J., … Schunemann, H. J. (2016). When and how to update systematic reviews: Consensus and checklist. *British Medical Journal, 354*, article 3507. ▶ https://doi.org/10.1136/bmj.i3507.

Garritty, C., Tsertsvadze, A., Tricco, A. C., Sampson, M., & Moher, D. (2010). Updating systematic reviews: An international survey. *PloS One, 5*, article 9914. ▶ https://doi.org/10.1371/journal. pone.0009914.

Gross, C. (2016). Scientific misconduct. *Annual Review of Psychology, 67*, 693–711. ▶ https://doi. org/10.1146/annurev-psych-122414-033437.

Higgins, J. P. T., Green, S., & Scholten, R. J. P. M. (2011). Maintaining reviews: Updates, amendments and feedback. In J. P. T. Higgins & S. Green (Eds.), *Cochrane handbook for systematic reviews of interventions. Version 5.1.0* [updated March 2011]. The Cochrane Collaboration. Retrieved from ▶ www.cochrane-handbook.org.

Hussinger, K., & Pellens, M. (2019). Guilt by association: How scientific misconduct harms prior collaborators. *Research Policy, 48*, 516–530. ▶ https://doi.org/10.1016/j.respol.2018.01.012.

Ioannidis, J. P. A. (2016). The mass production of redundant, misleading, and conflicted systematic reviews and meta-analyses. *The Milbank Quarterly, 94*, 485–514. ▶ https://doi.org/10.1111/1468-0009.12210.

John, L. K., Loewenstein, G., & Prelec, D. (2012). Measuring the prevalence of questionable research practices with incentives for truth telling. *Psychological Science, 23,* 524–532. ► https://doi.org/10.1177/0956797611430953.

Moher, D., Tsertsvadze, A., Tricco, A., Eccles, M., Grimshaw, J., Sampson, M., & Barrowman, N. (2008). When and how to update systematic reviews. *Cochrane Database of Systematic Reviews.* Retrieved from ► https://www.cochranelibrary.com/.

Pupovac, V., & Fanelli, D. (2015). Scientists admitting to plagiarism: A meta-analysis of surveys. *Science and Engineering Ethics, 21,* 1331–1352. ► https://doi.org/10.1007/s11948-014-9600-6.

Rees, R., & Oliver, S. (2017). Stakeholder perspectives and participation in reviews. In D. Gough, S. Oliver, & J. Thomas (Eds.), *An introduction to systematic reviews* (2nd ed., pp. 19–41). Thousand Oaks, CA: Sage.

Saunders, D. H., Greig, C. A., Young, A., & Mead, G. E. (2004). Physical fitness training for stroke patients. *Cochrane Database of Systematic Reviews.* ► https://doi.org/10.1002/14651858.cd003316.pub2.

Saunders, D. H., Sanderson, M., Hayes, S., Kilrane, M., Greig, C. A., Brazzelli, M., & Mead, G. E. (2016). Physical fitness training for stroke patients. *Cochrane Database of Systematic Reviews.* ► https://doi.org/10.1002/14651858.cd003316.pub6.

Shojania, K. G., Sampson, M., Ansari, M. T., Ji, J., Doucette, S., & Moher, D. (2007). How quickly do systematic reviews go out of date? A survival analysis. *Annals of Internal Medicine, 147,* 224–233. ► https://doi.org/10.7326/0003-4819-147-4-200708210-00179.

Simmonds, M., Salanti, G., McKenzie, J., & Elliott, J. (2017). Living systematic reviews: 3. Statistical methods for updating meta-analyses. *Journal of Clinical Epidemiology, 91,* 38–46. ► https://doi.org/10.1016/j.jclinepi.2017.08.008.

Thomas, J., Noel-Storr, A., Marshall, I., Wallace, B., McDonald, S., Mavergames, C., … Elliot, J. (2017). Living systematic reviews: 2. Combining human and machine effort. *Journal of Clinical Epidemiology, 91,* 31–37. ► https://doi.org/10.1016/j.jclinepi.2017.08.011.

Tod, D., & Edwards, C. (2015). A meta-analysis of the drive for muscularity's relationships with exercise behaviour, disordered eating, supplement consumption, and exercise dependence. *International Review of Sport and Exercise Psychology, 8,* 185–203. ► https://doi.org/10.1080/1750984X.2015.1052089.

United Kingdom Research Integrity Office. (n.d.). *Checklist for Researchers,* from ► http://ukrio.org/wp-content/uploads/UKRIO-Recommended-Checklist-for-Researchers.pdf.

University of Auckland. (2018). *Academics work together to uncover mass scientific fraud,* from ► https://www.auckland.ac.nz/en/about/news-events-and-notices/news/news-2018/08/academics-work-together-to-uncover-mass-scientific-fraud-.html.

12

Top Tips from the Experts

D. Tod, *Conducting Systematic Reviews in Sport, Exercise, and Physical Activity*,
https://doi.org/10.1007/978-3-030-12263-8_13

Learning Objective

After reading this chapter, you should be able to:
- Apply the top tips suggested by method experts and people publishing systematic reviews on sport, exercise, and physical activity topics.

Introduction

Systematic reviews help us advance knowledge in the sport, exercise, and physical activity domains, as well as assist practitioners in making evidence-based decisions. These types of reviews help ensure that the synthesis of research is methodical, rigorous, and transparent. Methodology has diversified in recent years as experts and researchers have explored ways to apply the review process to a range of evidence types and questions. The linear, aggregative, and quantitative procedures researchers use to meta-analyse randomized controlled trials are no longer the sole options available. Reviewers can tailor their efforts to answer whatever questions are meaningful and relevant to their fields of study.

Diversity in methodology, however, also means that inexperienced reviewers can feel uncertain about how to proceed. Their bewilderment might be compounded by the number of checklists, the plethora of acronyms, and the amount of jargon associated with systematic reviews. Inexperienced reviewers are likely to appreciate the words of advice and encouragement their mentors provide. For the final chapter, I invited method experts and researchers who have published reviews in the sport, exercise, and physical activity domains to offer advice on how to undertake these projects. I have arranged their quotes into themes to enhance your ability to remember them. I have also indicated a book or journal article the individuals have written so that you can follow up their work and learn from them.

Have a Clear Specific Question

13

> Never start off with the objective of just "reviewing the evidence". "Reviewing the evidence" is not on its own a useful objective. Instead, always work out where the genuine uncertainty is, and aim for your review to address that uncertainty. If you can't do that, the review risks being of little value. Mark Petticrew (Petticrew & Roberts, 2006; method expert and co-author of the book, *Systematic Reviews in the Social Sciences*)

Most people would likely agree with the above advice. The acronyms, such as PICO and SPIDER, can help individuals pinpoint uncertainty in their areas of study and formulate concrete specific review questions.

Develop Technical Expertise

> Essentially, performing meta-analyses affords rigorous scientific work to identify research articles and to extract the relevant data from the papers. Sound statistical knowledge is needed to analyse data and to derive appropriate conclusions. Meta-analyses are important research contributions because they provide statistically aggregated knowledge from several studies on a specific topic and they often

detect gaps in the literature. Urs Granacher (meta-analysis expert, see Gebel, Lesinski, Behm, & Granacher, 2018)

» Be as mindful of threats to quality of the data and interpretation as when doing empirical research. Keith George (meta-analysis expert, see Hulshof et al., 2019)

» Read and immerse yourself in all the guidance, textbooks and tool kits, but remember when you are doing your review to engage your own judgement and imagination. If you "bend the rules", simply explain and justify why you did things differently. Nicholas Mays (Pope, Mays, & Popay, 2007; method expert and co-author of the book, *Synthesizing Qualitative and Quantitative Health Evidence*)

» Enabling researchers to more objectively uncover some of the blind spots, scientific gaps and unintentional biases that exist in a body of work such that they can move an area forward with due diligence. This does require the researcher to be very switched onto sampling, contextual, cultural, and design-related study patterns emerging from the review that help reveal what future questions are hiding in plain sight! Chris Harwood (systematic review expert, see Harwood, Keegan, Smith, & Raine, 2015)

» Remember that we are always seeking "truth." The systematic review process and meta-analysis can be a blend of science and art, which will have tremendous impact on your field of study. With the rapid global publication rate, it is nearly impossible for practitioners and researchers to stay up to date on all of the current research. It is your job to synthesize an entire body of literature into one manuscript. The first steps of your systematic review are to outline your specific aim and refine your search strategy. We tell our students that, in many cases, the systematic review is used to identify gaps in the literature. The search for relevant articles is arguably the most important component of your project. If an article is not discovered, it will not be included. In the event that not much has been published on your topic, the systematic review could be very valuable in identifying potential directions for future research. Failing to include all relevant publications could potentially bias your results, especially when the cumulative body of research is small. Be thorough and exhaustive in your search. Michael Fedewa (meta-analysis expert, see Fedewa, Hathaway, Williams, & Schmidt, 2017)

Systematic reviews draw on a range of technical knowledge and skills to ensure the production of transparent and rigorous articles. Undertaking knowledge and skills audits can help identify competency gaps.

Ensure the Review Has Relevance

» What can I say!! I suppose my potentially irreverent advise to people attempting to systematically review current evidence on a topic is not to get hung up on technical 'rigour' - serious risk that the product will be characterised by intellectual 'mortice'. Seems to me at the end of a long career that an unhealthy obsession with review methods too often crowds out a focus on relevance and utility. Jennie Popay (Pope et al., 2007; method expert and co-author of the book, *Synthesizing Qualitative and Quantitative Health Evidence*)

» Don't do meta-analyses just because you can … the most important part of any research, including meta-analyses, is the rationale and sound underpinning to the question you are trying to answer. Keith George (meta-analysis expert, see Hulshof et al., 2019)

» A well conducted systematic review can provide a very useful roadmap for researchers and practitioners on the current literature in a particular area and clear directions for future research. They can be very useful for PhD students as a starting point for developing their thesis. However, it is important to identify if the systematic review is really needed given that there are many more appearing in the literature. Mike McGuigan (systematic review expert, see Douglas, Pearson, Ross, & McGuigan, 2017)

Reviews do not warrant publication because they are systematic or rigorous, but because they answer a relevant question that drives science forward, helps us make the world a better place, or both.

Plan the Review

» My advice would be to plan ahead! Write a good protocol, plan the analysis, and use a logic model to help ensure you have a coherent conceptual framework. Time invested in thinking things through properly at the outset will be more than repaid as you move through the review. James Thomas (method expert and co-author of *An Introduction to Systematic Reviews*, Gough, Oliver, & Thomas, 2017)

» After undertaking an initial scoping exercise of the literature, it is best to spend time refining the key concepts and variables of interest so that the take-home messages from the review are clear and concise. Furthermore, consider what other reviews (on similar topics) have been conducted and, even though the proposed manuscript will be newer (and hence pool the data from more up-to-date articles), researchers are advised to find a new angle (or angles), thus enabling a higher degree of novelty. Finally, make sure the data is checked and re-checked by several co-authors and, if more clarity is required, contact the authors of the original publication(s). Ajmol Ali (meta-analysis expert, Southward, Rutherfurd-Markwick, & Ali, 2018)

» Take the time at the start of your review to really understand and plan what you are trying to achieve and develop a suitable review question. By being as thorough and precise as you can be about the scope of your review and the methods you are going to use, you will save yourself a lot of time and difficult choices later on. For first time reviewers the rigorous methods can seem somewhat overwhelming. Do not be put off, however, by the jargon and technical processes common in systematic reviews or the volume of literature you may have to sift through, but use the guidelines and reference management software that are available to help you manage your review. Geoff Bates (systematic review expert, see Bates et al., in press)

» Take the time to carefully specify clear inclusion criteria. This is of great help in the process of selecting articles to include in the systematic review. Andreas Ivarsson (meta-analysis expert and statistical guru, see Ivarsson et al., 2017)

13

Avoid the temptation to start a review without a detailed protocol. If you must do something before you write a protocol, pilot test your ideas on a small sample of papers from beginning to end. The pilot test will help make sure the method works and you know how to drive the study.

Be Organized

» Be organized. Keep track of everything from why an article is not relevant to the page number where you found the effect size. Brooke Macnamara (meta-analysis expert, see Macnamara, Moreau, & Hambrick, 2016)

Organization would be one of my top tips given the amount of information generated during systematic reviews, and the level of detail expected in reporting standards.

Include Other People in the Process

» Build a good team and get constructive criticism and insight throughout the research process. Keith George (meta-analysis expert, see Hulshof et al., 2019)

» My top tip for reviewers would be to involve people with direct experience of the topic in the review planning, and in the reviewing if you can. Working with people who might benefit the review can help reviewers improve the external validity of their review questions, and improve their understanding of the topic. The process of identifying people will in itself be helpful in shaping the review. Are you doing this to help doctors, trainers, physiotherapists or athletes? Involving people who don't know about reviews can be challenging, but again, thinking about how to explain the review to someone outside of academia and talking to them about the planned work, will ultimately be helpful when it comes to writing up. Kristin Liabo (method expert, see Liabo, Gough, & Harden, 2017)

» When conducting systematic reviews my best advice is to always work in teams where several researchers are involved in the different steps. This will improve the quality of the work. Andreas Ivarsson (meta-analysis expert and statistical guru, see Ivarsson et al., 2017)

» Contact authors and leaders in the field for help. Keep in mind that conducting a meta-analysis does not make you an expert. The research world is small at the top, consult with the experts and other "truth-seekers" and invite them to collaborate. Many hands make light work. Michael Fedewa (meta-analysis expert, see Fedewa et al., 2017)

» For your first meta-analysis, try to have someone check every equation, method, adjustment, estimator choice, etc. Brooke Macnamara (meta-analysis expert, see Macnamara et al., 2016)

When the Beatles John Lennon and Paul McCartney wrote the song *Help!*, they had probably just being trying to do a systematic review.

Systematic Reviews Are Worthwhile and Satisfying Projects

» Systematic reviewing isn't as boring as you think – and it may even save lives. Helen Roberts (method expert and co-author of the book, *Systematic Reviews in the Social Sciences*, Petticrew & Roberts, 2006).

» Meta-analyses are a lot of work, but have an impact, so they are worth it. I get very excited each time I start a meta-analysis. At some point that fades and I think 'This is too all-consuming! I'm never doing a meta-analysis again.' Eventually it's published and that's very satisfying. Then I get an idea for a new one and go through the cycle again, but each time excitement is a little greater and the negative part is a bit lessened, so they get better and better. Brooke Macnamara (meta-analysis expert, see Macnamara et al., 2016)

» Systematic reviews represent the new 'gold standard' for scientific knowledge. Across virtually all disciplines of social sciences, medicine, education, and including sports and exercise science, the quantity of research findings have outpaced the ability of all but the most narrow of scholars to keep updated. Systematic reviews synthesize all available research to provide definitive statement of what is known, what is unknown, and where a field should next turn. Noel Card (meta-analysis expert and author of *Meta-Analysis for Social Science Research*, 2012)

» When someone asks me for advice about doing a systematic review, I tell them one thing: When you finish the review, you will say to yourself "I'm never doing one of those again." I know because that is what I have said to myself every time. But, when the pain and anguish of completing (publishing) the review fades, you start feeling ready to complete another one. Then when you finish the next review, you say …. and so the cycle continues. Nicholas Holt (systematic review expert, see Holt et al., 2017)

Experience can be a powerful teacher. The advice above has been forged from much effort and time spent applying the systematic review process to primary research. Further, the learning gained from experience is enhanced when combined with reflection, and I hope that you have the time to consider the words above from some highly experienced reviewers.

13

Summary

Keith George provided one quote I did not present above: "*Always write a meta-analysis with a gin and tonic in your hand.*" Keith's words remind us to keep systematic reviews in perspective and understand their role in science. Ben Goldacre's (2011, p. xi) following comment contains much truth that also applies to sport, exercise, and physical activity research: "*the notion of systematic review – looking at the totality of evidence – is quietly one of the most important innovations in medicine over the past 30 years.*" Systematic reviews help us advance knowledge, make suitable decisions about policy and practice, save and enhance lives, and improve society. But they do so only because of the high quality primary research that goes before them. Primary research and systematic reviews share a symbiotic relationship. Without primary research there is nothing to review. In turn, systematic reviews help to synthesize primary research so that individual studies can make their full contribution to human knowledge. No type of research, primary or secondary, qualitative or quantitative, empirical or review, provides complete answers to the difficult questions facing us as individuals and communities. Each design helps us in some way to organize ourselves and our societies so we can meet the challenges we face. Systematic reviews are a necessary part of the scientific industry, and I hope this book helps you succeed in undertaking reviews that allow you to offer new insights into our understanding of sport, exercise, and physical activity.

References

Bates, G., Begley, E., Tod, D., Jones, L., Leavey, C., & McVeigh, J. (in press). A systematic review investigating the behaviour change strategies in interventions to prevent misuse of anabolic steroids. *Journal of Health Psychology*. ▶ https://doi.org/10.1177/1359105317737607.

Card, N. A. (2012). *Applied meta-analysis for social science research*. New York, NY: Guilford.

Douglas, J., Pearson, S., Ross, A., & McGuigan, M. (2017). Chronic adaptations to eccentric training: A systematic review. *Sports Medicine, 47*, 917–941. ▶ https://doi.org/10.1007/s40279-016-0628-4.

Fedewa, M. V., Hathaway, E. D., Williams, T. D., & Schmidt, M. D. (2017). Effect of exercise training on non-exercise physical activity: A systematic review and meta-analysis of randomized controlled trials. *Sports Medicine, 47*, 1171–1182. ▶ https://doi.org/10.1007/s40279-016-0649-z.

Gebel, A., Lesinski, M., Behm, D. G., & Granacher, U. (2018). Effects and dose–response relationship of balance training on balance performance in youth: A systematic review and meta-analysis. *Sports Medicine, 48*, 2067–2089. ▶ https://doi.org/10.1007/s40279-018-0926-0.

Goldacre, B. (2011). Foreword. In I. Evans, H. Thornton, I. Chalmers, & P. Glasziou (Eds.), *Testing treatments: Better research for better healthcare* (2nd ed., pp. ix–xii). London, UK: Pinter & Martin Publishers.

Gough, D., Oliver, S., & Thomas, J. (2017). *An introduction to systematic reviews* (2nd ed.). Thousand Oaks, CA: Sage.

Harwood, C. G., Keegan, R. J., Smith, J. M. J., & Raine, A. S. (2015). A systematic review of the intrapersonal correlates of motivational climate perceptions in sport and physical activity. *Psychology of Sport and Exercise, 18*, 9–25. ▶ https://doi.org/10.1016/j.psychsport.2014.11.005.

Holt, N. L., Neely, K. C., Slater, L. G., Camiré, M., Côté, J., Fraser-Thomas, J., … Tamminen, K. A. (2017). A grounded theory of positive youth development through sport based on results from a qualitative meta-study. *International Review of Sport and Exercise Psychology, 10*, 1–49. ▶ https://doi.org/10.1080/1750984x.2016.1180704.

Hulshof, H. G., Eijsvogels, T. M. H., Kleinnibbelink, G., van Dijk, A. P., George, K. P., Oxborough, D. L., & Thijssen, D. H. J. (2019). Prognostic value of right ventricular longitudinal strain in patients with pulmonary hypertension: A systematic review and meta-analysis. *European Heart Journal—Cardiovascular Imaging, 20*, 475–484. ▶ https://doi.org/10.1093/ehjci/jey120.

Ivarsson, A., Johnson, U., Andersen, M. B., Tranaeus, U., Stenling, A., & Lindwall, M. (2017). Psychosocial factors and sport injuries: Meta-analyses for prediction and prevention. *Sports Medicine, 47*, 353–365. ▶ https://doi.org/10.1007/s40279-016-0578-x.

Liabo, K., Gough, D., & Harden, A. (2017). Developing justifiable evidence claims. In D. Gough, S. Oliver, & J. Thomas (Eds.), *An introduction to systematic reviews* (2nd ed., pp. 251–277). Thousand Oaks, CA: Sage.

Macnamara, B. N., Moreau, D., & Hambrick, D. Z. (2016). The relationship between deliberate practice and performance in sports: A meta-analysis. *Perspectives on Psychological Science, 11*, 333–350. ▶ https://doi.org/10.1177/1745691616635591.

Petticrew, M., & Roberts, H. (2006). *Systematic reviews in the social sciences: A practical guide*. Malden, MA: Blackwell.

Pope, C., Mays, N., & Popay, J. (2007). *Synthesizing qualitative and quantitative health evidence: A guide to methods*. Maidenhead, UK: Open University Press.

Southward, K., Rutherfurd-Markwick, K. J., & Ali, A. (2018). The effect of acute caffeine ingestion on endurance performance: A systematic review and meta-analysis. *Sports Medicine, 48,* 1913–1928.
  ▶ https://doi.org/10.1007/s40279-018-0939-8.

13

Supplementary Information

D. Tod, *Conducting Systematic Reviews in Sport, Exercise, and Physical Activity*,
https://doi.org/10.1007/978-3-030-12263-8

Index

A

Abstract stacking 48
Aggregative review 10, 45–46, 120–122, 154
AMSTAR-2 (A Measurement Tool to Assess System-
    atic Reviews) 134
Analysis definition 116
Archiving reviews 168–169

B

Black box review 3
Boolean operators 73

C

Cochrane, Archie 5
Cochrane Collaboration 5
Cognitive bias 103
Coherency 19, 89, 125
Configural review 10, 45–46, 122–124, 140–143,
    154–155
Control versus contrast groups 59–60
Critical appraisal 135–136, 100–112
– components 101
– conducting a critical appraisal (the 5 As) 106–107
– *critical appraisal nihilism* 112
– definition 100
– purposes 103–104
– qualitative research 107–110
– risk of bias versus quality 101–102

D

Data analysis 116–128
– aggregative approach 120–122
– configural approach 122–124
– generic procedure 118–119
– selecting a method 117–118
Data extraction 84–96
– codebook 87–88
– code sheet 87–88
– developing extraction tools 87–88
– documenting 90
– existing extraction tools 91
– information to extract 86–87

– principles 89
– purposes 84–85
– qualitative research 89–90
– verification 90
Deficiencies model of introductions 46–50
Disseminating review findings 148–161
– conference posters 157–158
– elements of high quality report (reporting stand-
    ards) 148–150
– oral presentations 157–158
– reasons 148
– stakeholders considerations 150–152
– writing reports 152–157

E

Economic evaluation review 7, 50–51
ESRC (Economic and Social Research Council) 150–
    152
Ethical considerations 164–166
– fabrication 164
– falsification 164
– plagiarism 164
– publication ethics 165–166
Evidence-based movement 5
Evidence table 91–93

G

GRADE (Grading of Recommendations, Assessment,
    Development, and Evaluations) 136–138, 144
– developing recommendations 139–140
– evidence profile 138
– procedure 136–138
– summary of findings 138
Grey (fugitive) literature 63, 74

I

Inclusion and exclusion criteria 56–65
– creating and using 61–62
– value 56–57
– writing 57–61
Introduction section 44–53
– deficiencies model 46–50
– objectives 44–45
– structure 44–50

L

Living reviews 171–172

M

Maintaining and update reviews 171–172
Mapping review 7
Measurement calibration 60
Meta-analysis 3, 7, 117–118, 120–122
Meta-ethnography 8
Meta-narrative 8, 117–118, 122–123
Meta-study 8
Mixed method review 124–127
– checklist 126–127
– coherence 125
– sequencing 125
– theoretical framework 126
– weighting 126

N

Narrative review 3

O

Olympic Games 10–12
Operational definition 56
Overviews 7

P

PICO (Participant, Intervention, Comparison, Outcomes) 22, 39, 57, 58, 63, 69, 87, 110, 143
Project management 24
– profiling 26–27
– The 4 Ps 24–25
Protocols 21–24
– benefits 21–22
– PRISMA (Preferred Reporting Items of Systematic
reviews and Meta-Analyses) protocol 20–24,
27–29
– PROSPERO protocol 21, 27–29
– registration 21–22
– structure 22
Publication ethics 165–166

R

RAMESES (Realist And Meta-narrative Evidence
Syntheses: Evolving Standards) 134

Realist synthesis 8, 123–124
Reporting standards 20, 21, 133–134, 148–150
Research design 104–106
– blind versus non-blind 106
– controlled versus uncontrolled 105
– cross-sectional versus longitudinal 105
– experimental versus descriptive 104–105
– prospective versus retrospective 105
– random versus non-random allocation 105
– random versus non-random selection 105
– within participant versus between participant 105
Research paradigms 108–109
– artistic 109
– critical change 109
– social constructivist 109
– traditional positivist 108
Review questions 32–41, 178
– factors influencing review questions 33–36
– mixed methods review questions 38
– qualitative review questions 37–38
– quantitative review questions 36, 36–37
– types of review questions 32
Risk of bias 101–102

S

Scientific misconduct 165
– motivation 165
– prevalence 165
Scoping review 7, 69–70
Searching the literature 68–81
– backward search 75
– boolean operators 73
– citation chasing 75
– contacting authors 75–76
– documentation 77–78
– document management 79
– electronic search 70–74
– filters 73
– forward search 75
– limits 74
– manual search 75
– MeSH (Medical Subject Headings) 72
– phases 68–69
– sampling frame 68
– scoping 69–70
– sensitive search 68
– specific search 68
Selective outcome reporting 21
Software and information tools 166–167
SPIDER (Sample, Phenomenon of Interest, Design,
Evaluation, Research type) 39, 63

STARLITE (Standards for Reporting Literature searches; Sampling strategy, Type of study, Approaches, Range of years, Limits, Inclusion and exclusions, Terms used, Electronic sources) 78
– stopping 78–79
– table of contents 75
– thesauri 71
– verification 76–77
Synthesis definition 4, 117
Systematic map 93–94
Systematic review
– assessing systematic reviews 132–145
– benefits 4
– collaboration 181
– definition 2–3
– disseminating findings 148–161
– diversity 7–8
– expertise 164, 178–179
– history 4–7
– knowledge contribution 45
– organization 181
– planning 180
– process (the 4 Cs) 16
– relevance 179
– top tips 178–183
Systematic review assessment 133–145
– configural reviews 140–143
– evidence synthesis 136–140
– GRADE 136–140
– included studies 135–136
– purposes 132–133

– review method focus 135
– review method rigour 133–134
– review method suitability 134–135

T

Thematic summary 122
Theoretical orientation 33–34, 126

U

Umbrella reviews 7
Updating and maintaining reviews 169–170
– frequency 170
– living reviews 171–172

V

Vote counting 120

W

Writing 152–157
– classic style 154–155
– plot 153–154
– practical style 154
– reflective style 154
– style 154

Printed in Great Britain
by Amazon

58515619R00111